Understanding Living Kidney Donation

The Best Treatment for Kidney Disease

Glenna Frey, MSN, APRN-CNS
Nephrology Nurse
Living Kidney Donor

An Unusual Copyright Page

~ because I want this information to be openly shared ~

Understanding Living Kidney Donation
The Best Treatment for Kidney Disease
Glenna Frey
Published 2025
Woodland Nook Press

Print ISBN: 979-8-234-16791-0

Printed in the United States of America

Funding for the book was generously provided by Kidney Donor Conversations, Inc.

Dedication

This book is dedicated to

Bob, Amanda, Sawyer, and Zora.

Thank you for sharing this

life with me.

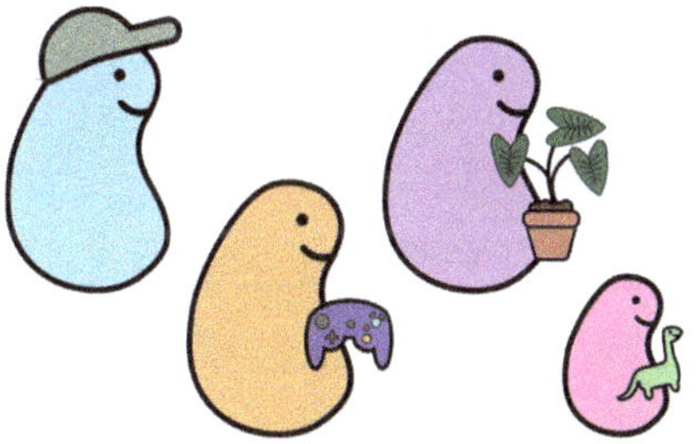

Be the Change
You Wish to See
in the World

~Gandhi

CONTENTS

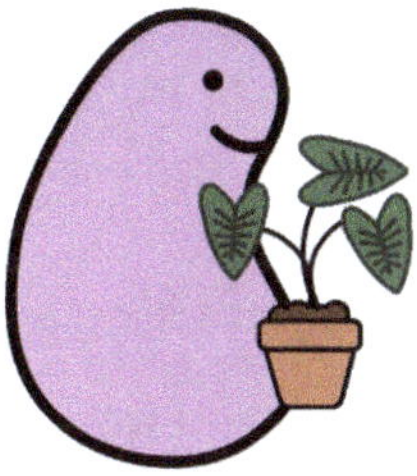

A Note From the Author's Daughter Amanda Frey, MA, LMFT, LPC, ACS

I'll start with saying that my mom is the most incredible person I know. 💖 (And as she reads this, I bet she's tearing up while also thinking that can't be true.) I could talk about how she's the best mom you could ask for, an amazing best friend, and an all-around impressive role model of a human. But this book is specifically about how much of her heart and soul she's put into her career, resulting in this book. I've learned so many amazing life lessons from her, either through watching her or talking to her, and having a career dedicated to something you love and care about is one of the huge things she's modeled for me. From nursing school, to every medical center she's worked at, to starting a Walk for Polycystic Kidney Disease, to co-founding a living kidney donation nonprofit, she puts her all into her work and commitments and love for the nephrology field. (A strange thing to love, in my opinion, but to each their own.)

My career, however, has nothing at all to do with nephrology. Because she showed me that an important part of work is loving what you do, I bailed on getting anywhere near a hospital and became a marriage & family therapist. And wow, do I love my job. In fact, it's the easiest part of my life; a luxurious statement I never actually aspired to claim. My job is full of analysis, vulnerability, compassion, education, laughter, tears, deep connection, and meaningful conversations. It's a challenge I look forward to, and that I feel shockingly competent at tackling. Every day I'm grateful to be allowed into my clients' lives, and humbled that I am able to help them grow and reach their goals.

How I became the co-founder of Kidney Donor Conversations (KDC) with my mom, as a therapist... I'm still not quite sure. Maybe it's because doing almost anything with her is fun and meaningful, and growing up around kidney disease taught me the importance of advocating in the nephrology field. But the more I think about it, the more I think it's really because I'm a therapist. Turns out my career has given me a lot of skills that have helped run the nonprofit. One of our big goals was to make living kidney donation an approachable topic that anyone can understand. Through work, I've become pretty skilled at communicating grad-school psychology concepts to any client in front of me. Which also means I can take grad-school nephrology concepts and make them easy to understand. I also have a slight eye for design and love being creative, both of which have helped make the nonprofit more fun and approachable. I also want to help make the world a better place, and saving lives through improved and increased kidney donations is an obvious way.

Throughout our time creating and running KDC, it became clear to me that my mom's whole life has led up to writing the book that you are about to read. You can read more about that in the Author's Note, but reflecting on it while living life with her has been wild. I think most people wonder what their life's book would be about, if they were to write one. Although on the surface this book isn't about my mom at all, it's an educational book about living kidney donation, so many of her life experiences and passions are fueling it. Without being a nephrology nurse, marrying into a family with kidney disease, and donating her own kidney, this book wouldn't exist. It took a million little things going exactly the right way, and if just one of them had been different she might not have written this book. This book is a physical cumulation of so many important moments and choices in my mom's life. How beautiful and deeply meaningful. Most people will never have something this tangible and heartfelt and helpful to represent their life and the paths they took.

So while you're reading this book, I hope you get more than just new information and a different perspective on living kidney donation. I hope you meet my mom on a deeper level, feel how much of her soul she put into writing it, and understand how this book is so much more than what's on the surface.

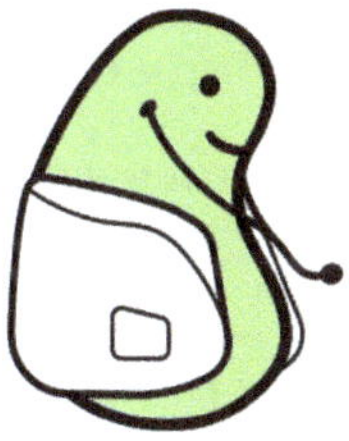

Foreword by Joshua Augustine, M.D.

After completing internal medicine residency training at Northwestern University in Chicago, IL, I had settled on pursuing further training in a nephrology (kidney medicine) fellowship. I had found during residency that treating and caring for patients with kidney disease was challenging but rewarding. I could function as a primary caregiver for these patients but with a focus on blood pressure, volume overload, acid base balance, and electrolyte management.

Transplantation was an obscure concept for me at that time. I was offered a fellowship at a prestigious program if I agreed to start the fellowship as a transplant trainee. I quickly declined, noting that I was not planning to focus on kidney transplantation. Little did I know that transplantation would consume my career for the next 20-plus years.

After initiating nephrology training at Cleveland Clinic, I quickly learned that outcomes were dismal in patients who remained tethered to dialysis machines. My first rotation on the kidney transplant service revealed patients who had hope and the promise of a healthier future. A patient waking up from anesthesia after receiving a living donor transplant stated that she felt a difference immediately, as the new kidney drained liters of urine and toxins from her body. I've heard similar patient comments now countless times over the years, and observed rapid changes in energy level, appetite, and even skin tone. One thing that puzzles me now is why transplantation, the optimal care for patients with kidney failure, is not practiced by all kidney medicine doctors. Many nephrologists make a career focusing on dialysis therapies while considering transplantation as a side option. I believe that we would have better outcomes and better patient (and doctor) satisfaction if transplantation was at the center of patient care.

One fascinating area of kidney transplantation, filled with ethical discussion and debate, is the evaluation and care of the living kidney donor. With the exception of a partial liver transplant donation, kidney transplant is unique in having the option for organ donation from a healthy living donor. Outcomes after living donor transplant are notably superior compared to deceased donor transplant. This is not surprising, as deceased donors typically suffer from chronic medical conditions contributing to death. Such conditions, if present, would often exclude living donor candidates from donating. Perhaps the most important concepts I have taken away from evaluating and caring for living donor candidates over the years are: A) the need to examine the donor's motivation and relationship to the recipient, and B) the need to recognize the detrimental effects suffered by the living donor candidate after being denied the opportunity to donate. Consider two cases:

Case I

A 19-year-old woman accompanied by her mom presented to the clinic as a potential donor to her brother, who suffered from congenital kidney disease. She was in ideal health physically with no medical contraindication for donation. During her evaluation, it was noted that her mother dominated the conversation and answered most of the questions asked by the healthcare team. After excluding the mom from the exam room, her daughter was first very quiet, then tearful, revealing that she was scared and felt like the process was moving very quickly. She was recommended not to donate at this time and was offered resources and counselling options. She appeared relieved that the process was put on hold.

Case 2

A woman in her sixties was turned down from donation initially because her labwork found her to be "pre-diabetic." She was obese and had high cholesterol. She intended to donate to her husband, who had started hemodialysis three months prior and since then had already had admissions to the hospital for a catheter-associated bloodstream infection and congestive heart failure. Her relationship to her husband had turned from a partner to a caregiver, and she had to take extensive time away from work to care for him at home. She knew that his health and independence could be improved with a living donor transplant. The woman was devastated when she was told she was not a donor candidate, and wisely sought a second opinion from another transplant center. Rather than just checking a box, the second center had in-depth discussions, which included social work and a bioethics team. It was noted that the patient had purposefully lost close to 15 pounds in weight, consistent with her motivation to donate. It was reasoned that if she progressed to full diabetes (less likely with weight loss), it would take another 15 to 20 years to develop diabetic-related kidney disease, at which point she would be in her eighties or older. The bioethics team recognized her motivation and discussed the need for informed consent, recognizing that she may have more risk than a younger and healthier donor. She was carefully consented and approved for donation. Two years after donating, the woman and her husband traveled to Italy and toured the Tuscany region. He was instructed only to make sure he had all his medicines packed prior to travel, to drink plenty of sterile water, and to wear potent sunscreen to protect against the Tuscan sun. The wife was grateful for the opportunity to improve her husband's health, as well as her quality of life, as she transitioned back into a partner role with her husband.

The book herein is an extremely useful guide written by Glenna Frey, MSN, APRN-CNS. Glenna offers a unique perspective as a long-time caregiver in nephrology, as a caregiver and partner at home supporting a loved one with kidney disease, and as a living kidney donor who has witnessed first-hand the process of donor evaluation, approval, surgery, and recovery. Who better to help the reader to navigate the incredibly intricate process of living kidney donation? Glenna has been a champion of living donation in her community and elsewhere for years. Clearly, like the vast majority of kidney donors, she views the donation process as challenging but positive and rewarding, with the chance to give a loved one or even a stranger better health and longevity. I found this book to be insightful, practical, and comprehensive, all with an "insider's view" from somebody who has been there.

There Are Many Kidneys

There are many kidneys.
Most people have two and only need one.

There are many resources.

~ to support finding living donor transplants for those with kidney disease.

~ to support those healthy enough and brave enough to donate a kidney.

There are many ways to improve efforts to discover more kidney donors.

Millions of healthy adults who have a kidney that could be donated.

An integrated system could exist for living donors similar to the system for deceased donors.

There are many resources and enough kidneys when we choose to break the silence and be a part of the change.

I cannot change the world
but I can cast a stone to
create many ripples.

~Mother Teresa

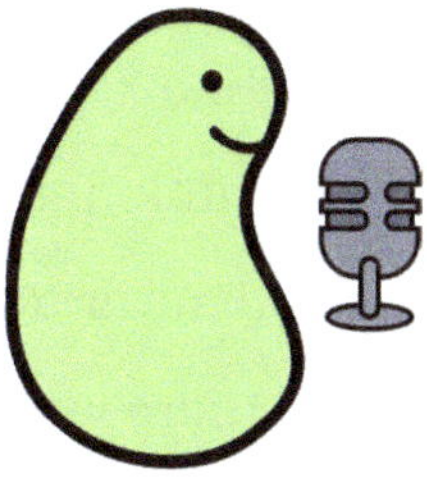

INTRODUCTION

Before that fall day in 2015, I had been waiting for the right time to fulfill my dream of being a living kidney donor. But I struggled with not knowing exactly when my husband might need a kidney transplant again. I had recently celebrated my 57th birthday. As I was standing in our dining room, my husband casually smiled and said to me, "You are getting older." That stung. I was only six months older than him, so I snidely replied, "So are you. So what?" Then what he said brought chills to my body and sparked a fire inside of me. He told me that since his current kidney was working so well, if I wanted to donate my kidney, I shouldn't wait until he needed it ... maybe I should donate sooner rather than later. I had been saving one of my kidneys for him for over 13 years. I immediately knew deep in my soul that it was finally time to start the process of donating my kidney. But not to him.

As a nephrology nurse with over 40 years of experience, I thought I knew everything about kidney donation. I was wrong. Prior to donating, I had never talked to a living donor about the entire process, and there was much for me to learn. That is why my daughter, Amanda, encouraged me to write this book. It is like a window looking into the living kidney donation experience. I want this topic to be less mysterious and more accessible for anyone to discuss.

The plight of the kidney donor is not always easy. It can be difficult, filled with stress, worry, and fear of the unknown. Afterward, however, almost all donors say they would do it again. Like me, some wish they had more kidneys to give and wish we could help more people.

Common Concerns About Living Kidney Donation

When talking with people about living kidney donation, it is common to hear responses like:

- I didn't know you could donate a kidney. If we have two kidneys, don't we need both?
- I didn't realize life on dialysis was so shitty.
- I would donate if it would save someone's life.
- I want to help, but ...
    - I am too old
    - I can't afford the time off work.

- I don't know if I'm healthy enough.
- What if one of my children needs a kidney later?
- What if I get kidney disease and may need my other kidney?
- I'm afraid of surgery and maybe dying. My family needs me.
- My family and friends will think I'm crazy if I have an unnecessary surgery.
- I can't afford to pay someone else to care for my children (or my aging parents) while I recover.

Most living kidney donors write books about their own personal donation process. But this book reveals a broader perspective for donors and recipients including why a living kidney transplant is best, the ways to donate a kidney, and the stages of living kidney donation.

Exploring these concerns may alleviate fears and enhance understanding of living kidney donation.

Why This Book About Living Kidney Donation?

While most living donors write books about their personal donation process, this book provides a broader perspective beyond my personal experience. Over the next 13 chapters, these topics will be explored:

- Facts about organ donation and why registering to be an organ donor is not enough
- Benefits of a living kidney donor transplant
- Ways to donate a kidney
- Benefits and risks of living donation
- Stages of living kidney donation

I have experience in caring for patients with kidney disease, including those undergoing hemodialysis, peritoneal dialysis, end-of-life care, and kidney transplants. Many of my family members have had kidney disease, undergone dialysis, and received living donor kidney transplants. Other family members donated their kidney. I have intimately seen the struggles and challenges that kidney disease imposes on people's lives. That's why I donated my kidney in 2017 to a complete stranger—to help someone live a happier, healthier life free from dialysis. I was also a voucher donor. My husband and daughter have vouchers to be matched with a kidney in the future if they develop kidney failure. (Refer to the chapter "Ways to Donate a Kidney" for more information about voucher programs.)

Donating my kidney has changed the trajectory of my life. I have been fulfilled in more ways than I can put into words. I have been blessed to meet numerous other donors, people with kidney disease, and professionals in kidney-related organizations across the country. In 2018, my daughter, Amanda Frey, and I co-founded the nonprofit Kidney Donor Conversations to provide education and support for living kidney donation. After years of giving living kidney donation presentations, discussions with donors, and talking with the public, it was time to share this information through a book to reach more people. My inside view and unique perspective provide details and guidance that may not be received from other healthcare professionals. There has been a call to enhance education about living kidney donation to supplement the information provided by transplant centers. This is an effort to address that need.

Some might question why the book is titled *Understanding Living Kidney Donation: The Best Treatment for Kidney Disease* when it is technically the best treatment for kidney failure. The intent is to encourage discussions about living kidney donation much earlier in the disease process, well before kidney failure occurs.

What This Book Is and Isn't

This book discusses adult kidney transplants and living kidney donation in the United States. There are variations in transplant center policies across the country, so my goal is to provide general information about the kidney transplant system. This work is not specific to a center and does not represent any particular program. I have a basic assumption that transplant centers will appropriately screen any potential donor without bias. That means I trust the process to work as it was designed. The information on living kidney donation is based on my experience and current evidence.

This book is not intended to:

- Provide medical advice
- Cover every aspect of living donation
- Determine specific eligibility for kidney donation
- Discuss all the evaluation tests required before donation

Information changes quickly! I have done my best to provide relevant and current information and resources. It may be helpful to visit websites or contact organizations directly to ensure the information in this book is still accurate.

The terms "donor" and "potential donor" are used interchangeably for ease of reading. No one is a kidney donor until they have actually undergone surgery to remove their kidney.

Most people are born with two kidneys but need only one to lead a healthy life. Let's normalize the idea that living kidney donation is an option for many adults. Let's provide more resources and have more conversations about living kidney donation.

The Kidney Dilemma

For eight years, I worked in outpatient cancer centers providing complementary therapies for people going through radiation and chemotherapy. I straddled the two worlds of kidney disease and cancer, noticing many differences. I see beautiful cancer centers being built with large window views to gardens to enjoy during treatment. The dialysis units often have few windows or high windows without a pleasant view. Cancer is known to be overdiagnosed at early stages. The best treatment is provided through radiation, chemotherapy, and immunotherapy. Those with cancer are often still aggressively treated until they die in Stage 4. Kidney disease is underdiagnosed throughout all stages, and few people are provided the best treatment—a living donor transplant. Screening for cancer is a high priority, integrated into the medical system, and screening for kidney disease is often ignored and rarely discussed. For further reading on the issue of cancer overdiagnosis, see Srivastava et al., 2019.

I am shocked at the discrepancy in the number of resources, fundraising events, emotional support, financial support, publicity, etc. that are provided on behalf of people with cancer compared to those with kidney disease, and especially to those on dialysis. There are about **35.5 million** people in the U.S. with kidney disease, or 1 in 7 people. Of those, 9 in 10 adults don't even know they have chronic kidney disease. Currently, approximately $18.00 is spent per kidney patient for research, compared to $305 per cancer patient. And there are fewer people with cancer, at about **18 million.** Kidney disease affects more people and is provided with fewer resources.

The Best Treatment for Kidney Failure

Currently, the best treatment for most people in kidney failure is a living donor kidney transplant. Unfortunately, this is the least discussed, least researched, and least funded treatment. Instead, our society, healthcare system, and healthcare providers are much more likely to focus on dialysis. Over 80% of people newly diagnosed with end-stage kidney disease begin with dialysis, even though it is better to get a kidney transplant first before ever starting dialysis (this will be discussed in more detail later). Since about 90% of people with chronic kidney disease (CKD) don't know they have it, there is typically denial, stress, and an urgent need to keep them alive, so all the treatment options are not thoroughly explored. There is not a thoughtful and comprehensive plan for what might be best for the person in regard to family life, work, social support, long-term goals, or personal values. Decisions have to be made under significant time constraints in very high-stress situations. Unfortunately, people cannot receive a transplanted kidney quickly. Typically, it takes months to complete the evaluation to see if they are healthy enough for a kidney transplant. And it may take years of waiting to receive a kidney from a deceased donor. This puts most patients in the position of choosing a quick treatment (dialysis), not the best treatment (living kidney transplant).Society's lack of focus on kidney disease often means people progress into kidney failure swiftly (chronic kidney disease Stage 5) and must urgently begin dialysis while they are in the hospital and very sick. (Refer to Appendix 1, "Chronic Kidney Disease Stages.")

Is There a Better Way?

People with kidney disease who begin planning early in the process have the best outcomes. Ideally, this planning would take place before or during chronic kidney disease Stage 4. This allows time for education, family discussion, exploring values, identifying priorities, and planning in advance. This also allows time to grieve the loss of kidney function and the other consequences that may come with it. The best outcomes are realized when a living donor transplant is obtained before going on dialysis. Mortality rates vary depending on the kidney failure treatment. After one year of dialysis, the mortality rate is 15% to 20%, with a five-year survival rate of less than 50%. In contrast, those who receive transplants have a five-year survival rate of about 80%. For anyone already on dialysis, the sooner they can be transplanted, the better.

The Organ Procurement and Transplantation Network clearly defines those with CKD who should be referred for transplant: "All patients with advanced CKD should be considered for transplant evaluation. The medical literature clearly demonstrates that kidney transplant is a superior form of kidney replacement therapy compared to dialysis. As such, referral to transplant should be the default care plan for CKD patients. There are no strict criteria for referral, but most patients with stage 4-5 CKD are appropriate for referral." Even with these very clear guidelines from a respected organization, only 16% to 34% of people are referred.

Everyone seems to understand the severity of cancer, and there seems to be a lack of similar understanding and empathy for those with kidney disease. The mean survival for people who start dialysis is three years. Survival is lower than for those who have solid organ cancer.

After a cancer diagnosis, people are offered the best radiation and chemotherapy treatment. They are not required to find the radiation machine or the medications. But those who want the best treatment for kidney disease must find their own treatment: someone willing to donate a kidney while alive. There is not a single streamlined system to supply patients with living kidney transplants. The medical system easily provides treatment for other diseases such as medications, artificial joints, heart valves, blood, etc. without the sick patients needing to source these items themselves.

When a bone marrow transplant is needed, there is a registry that will find a match with access to more than 39 million potential bone marrow donors. The NMDP (formerly known as the National Marrow Donor Program and Be the Match program) website states:

> "For patients diagnosed with leukemia, lymphoma and other life-threatening diseases, a bone marrow or cord blood transplant may be their best or only hope for a cure. Yet 70% of patients who need a transplant do not have a fully matched donor in their family. They depend on NMDP and our supporters to find a match to save their life. We also provide one-on-one support to patients and their families throughout the transplant journey. For more than 35 years, we've managed the most diverse blood stem cell registry in the world—and

the only one that's federally funded and Congressionally authorized."

Solid organ transplants and bone marrow transplants have different processes. However, there could be a single federally funded system like this for living kidney donors. Potential kidney donors could easily get started by filling out a health form and giving a cheek swab sample online or at a health fair. They could then be registered for further testing, with the possibility of being matched to someone needing a kidney transplant. Making the initial steps more accessible and raising awareness could lead to more living donors. There has to be a better way to help the 90,000 people on the kidney transplant waiting list than what we are currently providing.

Questions That Need Answers

Here are some questions that would benefit the kidney community if answered:

- What are the most effective methods to inform the public about the need for more funding, screening, and awareness for kidney disease?
- How can we best provide resources for individuals with kidney failure who need a living kidney transplant?

- What are the most effective ways to convey that a kidney from a living donor lasts longer than one from a deceased donor?
- How can we best educate, streamline, and support those who are inspired to donate?

It is time to break the culture of silence and offer resources and support that are easy to access so those with kidney disease receive the best treatment: a living donor transplant.

Myths are the instruments by which we continually struggle to make our experience intelligible to ourselves.

~Adrienne Rich

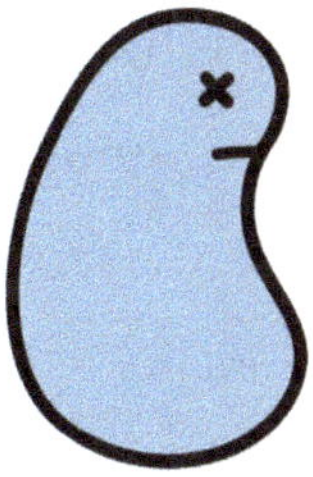

The Big Organ Donation Myth

Breaking the silence around living kidney donation starts with understanding the myth of organ donation from deceased donors. This chapter reveals why more living donors are needed and why deceased donors are not filling the huge gap for those on the kidney transplant waiting list.

There is not a kidney shortage; there is a kidney *allocation* crisis. There are around 90,000 people on the kidney transplant waiting list. There are 27.3 million healthy adults in the U.S. with a kidney that could be donated. That means there are enough kidneys. We need a better system that supports discovering more living donors.

Deceased Organ Donation

The typical solution to the long transplant waiting list is to get more people to register to be an organ donor at death. This strategy has not worked. **Less than 1% of the people who are registered as deceased organ donors will ever donate.**

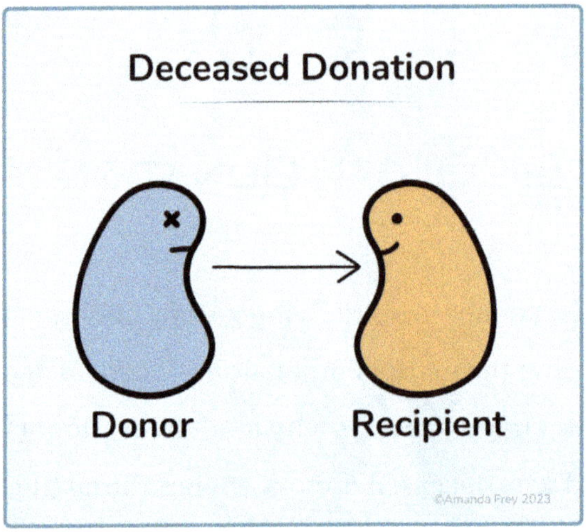

Registering to be an organ donor after death does not guarantee your organs will be donated. There are three main reasons why organ donation may not happen when someone dies:

1. They don't die in "the right way."

   Typically, to be a deceased donor, one must be pronounced brain dead without damage to other organs. Some examples of injuries that may cause brain death are an automobile accident, motorcycle accident, drowning, or drug overdose. These situations involve sudden, traumatic incidents where rescue efforts have taken place, but the individual sustains a severe neurological injury. They are in an intensive care unit on a mechanical ventilator which supports sending oxygen to their lungs and organs. That is a very specific way to die. Cardiac death can also result in organ donation; however, it is not as common as a neurologic event leading to brain death.

Most of us will die in other ways, as a result of a chronic disease (heart, lung, kidney, stroke, cancer, diabetes, etc.) or a serious infection in the hospital. Others will die in a nursing home, with hospice care or at home. Some people imagine dying peacefully in their sleep in their nineties. However, these situations do **not** result in organ donation. In spite of our best intentions, most of us will never be organ donors when we die because of *how* we die.

2. The organs aren't "healthy enough."

   According to Organ Procurement & Transplantation Network (OPTN) policies, upon death, the body and organs must be healthy enough to be transplanted to someone else. This criteria is different from living kidney donation. Some examples of general situations when kidney donation is **not** possible at death include:

- Greater than 70 years old
    - Cancer:
    - Current cancer (does not include non-melanoma skin cancers such as basal cell and squamous cell and primary brain tumors without metastatic disease)
    - Prior cancer with current metastatic disease
    - A history of melanoma
    - Leukemia, Hodgkin's disease, lymphoma, multiple myeloma
- No discernible cause of death
- Age 50–69 years with a history of type 1 diabetes for more than 20 years
- Polycystic kidney disease
- Glomerulosclerosis
- Chronic kidney failure
- No urine output for 24 hours or longer
- Active infections:
    - It is important to note that there are situations when organs from HIV positive donors can be transplanted. Details can be found in the HIV Organ Policy Equity (HOPE) Act.
    - There are also situations when organs from hepatitis B or hepatitis C positive donors can be transplanted.

3. The family does not give "consent."

Even though laws allow "first person consent" for organ donation, in many situations, the family must consent to donating the organs of someone who is brain dead. It can be very stressful and emotional for families when a loved one is suddenly injured and taken to the intensive care unit. In one study, 48% of Organ Procurement Organizations ranked the impact on the deceased family as the most important factor for consent, whereas only 12% believed the deceased's wishes were a higher priority. Families often don't discuss death and organ donation beforehand, so a person's wishes about donating organs after a tragic death may not be known to their next-of-kin. Even if wishes are known, whoever is designated to make decisions may not choose to donate.

Deceased donation provides people with more than just kidneys. Other solid organs such as heart, lung, pancreas, and liver (living liver and living uterus donation are also options) can be transplanted. These organs save many lives. It may be hard to believe, but even when someone donates their organs after death, some of their usable organs get thrown away instead of transplanted each year. In 2016, over 3,000 kidneys of deceased donors were discarded. Some discarded organs were too damaged to use. But other usable organs, like kidneys lost during transport, could have been transplanted instead of thrown away. The 57 Organ Procurement Organizations across the United States, which are contracted by the federal government to facilitate the deceased organ donation process, have historically operated with minimal oversight. These organizations are responsible for approaching families about donation, overseeing the donor's care until surgery, matching organs with recipients, coordinating surgery schedules, and transporting organs. Kidneys can only be out of the body for up to 36 hours before needing to be transplanted. If the organ procurement agencies are not communicating efficiently with the transplant team, or there are delays in transportation, or each step is not coordinated in a timely manner, organs may be thrown away. More people could be receiving life-saving organs if improvements were made in inefficient systems.

In 2022, Donate Life America launched the National Donate Life Living Donor Registry. People between the ages of 18–65 who register to be an organ donor will also be offered to register their interest in being a living kidney donor. A pilot program began in December 2021 in Texas. This program has not expanded and is not easily accessed by the general public because it is buried within the deceased donor registration process. A better model would be one that allows individuals to easily complete a health questionnaire, provide a cheek swab, then start the process to be a living donor. This could be done at health fairs, community events, hospitals, etc. A single, national registry for living donors could be the most efficient way to provide this service to the public. Currently there are multiple registries that are not linked. There is not one place for all potential donors to be registered.

Insights for the Chapter: The Big Organ Donation Myth

- Organ donation cannot be guaranteed at death, even if you are registered to donate your organs.
- Less than 1% of registered donors will be able to donate organs at death.
- You are not an organ donor until you actually donate an organ.

Only if we understand can we care.

Only if we care will we help.

~Jane Goodall

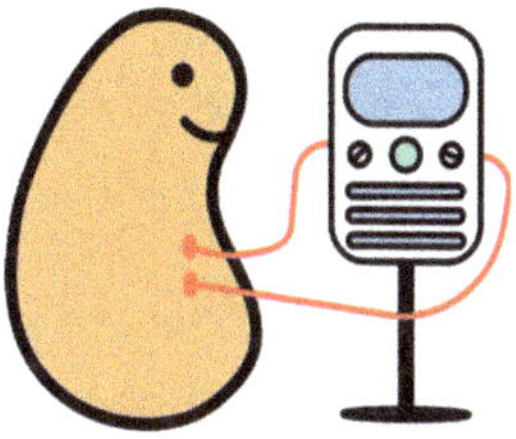

Treatments for Kidney Failure: The Worst and the Best

Many people lack awareness or understanding of how kidneys function. Those with healthy kidneys may not think about them at all. Those on dialysis may not talk with doctors or dialysis staff about getting a healthy kidney (transplant). Those waiting for a kidney transplant might not care if the kidney comes from someone who is alive or someone who has died. But depending on the quality of the kidney, people may experience different health outcomes.

It's important to learn about kidneys, kidney disease, dialysis, and how transplants from living and deceased donors differ. Once these concepts are understood, the value of receiving a kidney from a living donor becomes clearer.

Kidneys

Most people have two bean-shaped kidneys, about the size of a fist, that are located just below the rib cage, one on each side of the spine. Kidneys filter waste, drugs, and fluid from the blood, which are then removed as urine. They help maintain a balance of minerals such as sodium, calcium, phosphorus, and potassium in the blood. Without this balance, nerves, muscles, and other tissues in the body may not work normally. Kidneys also make hormones that help:

- control blood pressure
- make red blood cells
- keep bones strong and healthy

Chronic kidney disease is a slow, gradual loss of normal kidney function that affects both kidneys. The five chronic kidney disease stages reflect this loss of function (refer to table "Chronic Kidney Disease" in the Introduction). As kidney function severely declines, waste products, excess fluid, and electrolytes build up in the body, while other vital kidney functions diminish. The kidneys can't do their job anymore. People get very sick and will eventually die without treatment.

The main causes of kidney disease are diabetes, high blood pressure, inflammation in the kidneys (such as glomerulonephritis, interstitial nephritis, lupus, and Alport syndrome), stones, infections, medications, and genetic kidney diseases (such as polycystic kidney disease, or PKD). When kidney failure (chronic kidney disease Stage 5) is reached, a kidney transplant or dialysis is needed to keep people alive.

There's a misconception that having more kidneys leads to better health. This is incorrect. Chronic kidney disease doesn't progress by damaging one kidney and then the other. Instead, both kidneys are affected. If you have chronic kidney disease, **both kidneys are diseased.**

Dialysis

Dialysis is a method used to treat chronic kidney failure by cleaning the blood. But this is done less effectively and is a poor substitute for a healthy kidney. It only does about 5–15% of the job that one good kidney can do. Over time, kidneys stop doing other important jobs too. They can't make hormones that control blood pressure, help make red blood cells, or keep bones strong. Dialysis places an abnormal stress on the body. That is why most people on dialysis do not feel well, have little energy, have a low quality of life, and die early. People on dialysis have a cardiovascular risk 10 to 20 times higher than that of people who are not on dialysis.

Instead of being healthy, active, and fully engaged in life, living on dialysis for most people is more like Stage 4 cancer. Some people do not like the comparison of end-stage kidney disease with end-stage cancer, but the disease course can be similar, and often people are just a few steps away from death. Dialysis is not a cure. Dialysis leads to a gradual decline in health, making it a poor substitute for a healthy kidney. The five-year survival rate for people on dialysis is about 38%, and the ten-year survival rate is approximately 16%. The typical life expectancy for a person receiving dialysis treatment ranges from 5 to 10 years. Therefore, very few people live over 20 years on dialysis.

The two main types of dialysis are hemodialysis and peritoneal dialysis. Hemodialysis takes the blood out of the body through special tubes, filters the blood, and returns it. A special access is needed to get the blood out so it can be filtered. This is done either through a soft plastic tube called a catheter or a surgery in the arm called a fistula. Hemodialysis typically occurs three times a week in an outpatient facility. Each session takes about four hours sitting in a chair. People can also learn to perform hemodialysis treatments on themselves at home, several days a week.

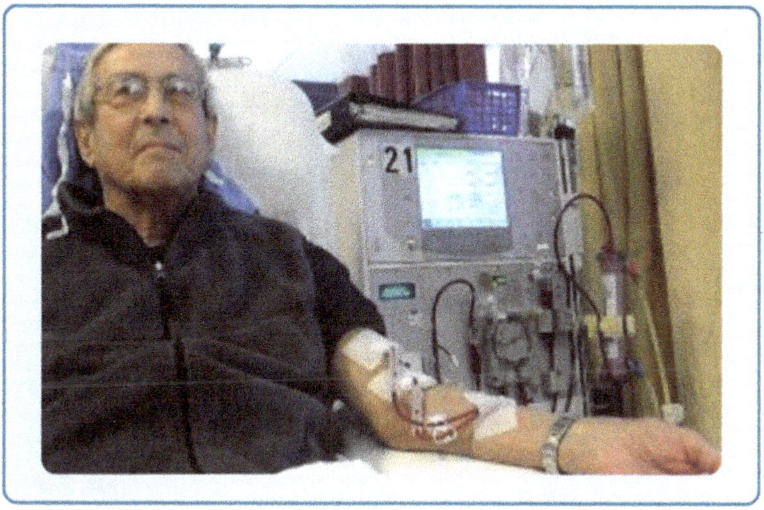

Man Receiving Hemodialysis (Raymond)

Peritoneal dialysis takes a sterile fluid that flows by gravity through a tube that enters the space in the abdomen called the peritoneum. About two liters of fluid goes in, stays there for several hours, then is drained out. The waste from the blood goes into the fluid and is later removed and discarded. New, fresh fluid is then allowed to enter the peritoneum, and the cycle continues. Peritoneal dialysis is done every day, as the sterile fluid is cycled in and the soiled fluid is cycled out to clean the blood. The timeframe for the cycles can be flexible. Some choose to provide the dialysis during the day. Others may choose overnight, using a machine called a cycler.

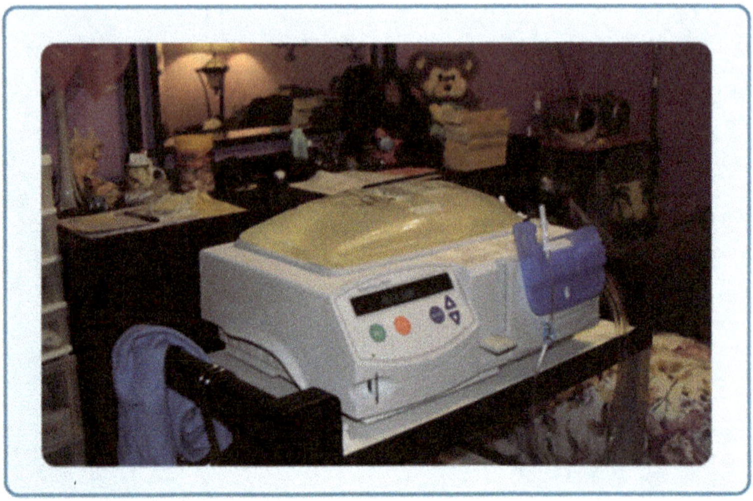

Peritoneal Dialysis Cycler (Flores)

Transplant

A kidney transplant is the best available treatment for kidney failure. A healthy kidney is connected to the blood vessels and bladder to take over the work of the diseased kidneys.

Compared to dialysis, a kidney transplant can provide:

- Better quality of life
- More free time
- More stable blood pressure, hormone, and electrolyte levels
- Higher rates of employment
- Decrease in symptoms

- Longer life
- Less use of healthcare resources

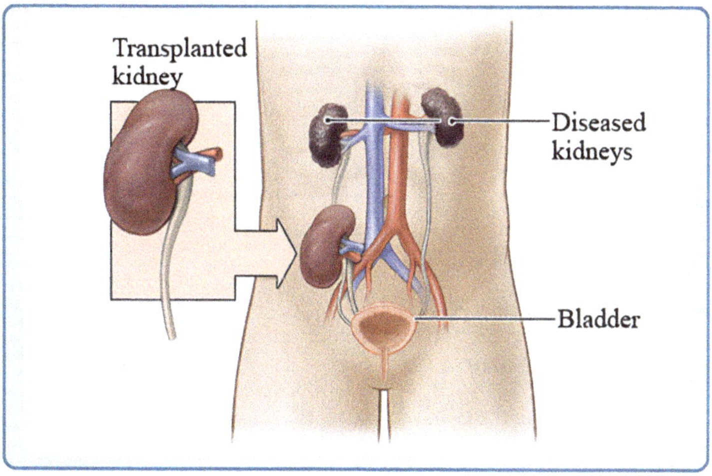

Location of Transplanted Kidney (Mayo)

If individuals meet the criteria for a kidney transplant, transplant centers add them to the deceased donor waiting list. Unfortunately, there aren't enough deceased donors for the 90,000 people on the waiting list. In 2023:

- 27,000 people received a kidney
    - Three-fourths were from deceased donors
    - One-fourth were from living donors
- 63,000 people did **not** get a kidney
    - 5,000 died waiting for a kidney

It is best if a transplant can be received before starting dialysis. This is called a preemptive transplant. Given that the average waiting time for a deceased kidney is five years or more, and life expectancy on dialysis is 5–10 years, many people will die waiting for a transplant. Most people who get kidney failure without planning for a transplant will start dialysis and die while on it. This is a hard truth that isn't often discussed.

The average life expectancy of a 55-year-old:

- *on dialysis is 5 years*
- *with a kidney transplant is 15 years*

Many believe that receiving a kidney from a deceased donor is equivalent to getting one from a living donor. However, there are important differences between these two types of kidney transplants.

A deceased donor transplant:

- Takes an average of five years to get a kidney
- May not work right away, which is called delayed graft function; some people will need dialysis after transplant for a short time while waiting for the kidney to start working
- Lasts 10–15 years

A living donor kidney transplant:

- Has less waiting time (often less than a year, or the time it takes for a living donor to be accepted to donate)
- Will almost always start working immediately
- Lasts 15–20 years
- Recipients experience better cognitive outcomes

It is often less effort to remain on dialysis and wait for a kidney from a deceased donor than to actively seek a living donor. The responsibility to find a living donor typically falls on the person needing a kidney. This process involves discussing kidney disease, life on dialysis, the risk of death, and the benefits of a living donor transplant with family, friends, or even strangers. These conversations can be challenging and may involve financial costs for advertising through websites, t-shirts, signs, or billboards. Some organizations offer social media platforms to help find donors, but even with multiple potential donors, there is no guarantee that any will be suitable for donation. Finding a living kidney donor is especially difficult for those who are very sick on dialysis, as it requires considerable effort, time, and support.

Compounding this challenge are significant disparities in kidney care among different racial groups. Black and African American individuals experience kidney failure more than three times as often as white individuals, while Hispanic and

Latino individuals experience it 1.3 times more frequently. Contributing factors include higher rates of high blood pressure, diabetes, obesity, and heart problems among people of color, as well as systemic barriers to accessing quality healthcare. Despite representing only 13.5% of the population, Black and African American individuals make up more than 35% of dialysis patients. They are also less likely to be placed on the transplant waiting list, face longer wait times, and have a lower likelihood of receiving a living donor transplant. These disparities have persisted for many years, underscoring the need for equitable kidney care for all.

High Cost of Dialysis and the Deceased Donor System

Due to regional variations, annual fluctuations, inflation, and differing sources of cost estimates, finding and interpreting the complex cost figures for dialysis and kidney transplants can be challenging. Here are some interesting cost estimates to consider.

People with a kidney transplant not only live longer and report a higher quality of life, but they cost the government and taxpayers less money than those on dialysis. In 2019, Medicare spending for hemodialysis was the most expensive treatment for end-stage kidney disease, costing $94,608 per person annually. Peritoneal dialysis cost $81,091 per person annually, while a kidney transplant was the least expensive treatment at $38,863 per person annually.

Dialysis creates a significant environmental burden. An average of 100,000 people per year are on in-center dialysis. Each person on hemodialysis uses over 5,000 gallons of quality water annually. The electricity consumed for one treatment is equivalent to the daily use of an average household. Each dialysis treatment generates up to 18 pounds of plastic and cardboard waste. Additionally, dialysis contributes to massive carbon dioxide emissions through water, energy, consumables usage, and transportation for staff and patients. Hemodialysis patients have more than seven times the carbon footprint of the average person. Peritoneal dialysis (PD) uses significantly less power and water compared to hemodialysis. It also produces less waste per treatment, but because PD is a daily therapy, the annual waste generation per patient is higher. Most of the waste from PD consists of plastic, including dialysate bags, outer packaging, and tubing. Receiving a kidney transplant eliminates much of this environmental waste burden.

In 2015, the cost of a kidney transplant for the first year was about $145,000. These costs can vary depending on the geographic location of the transplant center, the type of insurance coverage, and the individual patient's medical condition. This includes pre-transplant evaluation, hospitalization for the transplant surgery, transplant medications, and follow-up care. After the first year, medical costs were about $32,000 annually.

Living donor kidney transplant costs are lower than deceased donor costs, which are not only higher but are also rising. The Organ Procurement Organizations (OPOs) have operational costs to maintain buildings, staff, computer systems, and the day-to-day business related to the deceased donation process and the many people on the waiting list. These resources are not used to help people obtain a living donor transplant. On average, the cost to recover a deceased donor kidney in the United States is $36,000. Keeping patients on the transplant waiting list is also costly, requiring many medical tests each year, with an average wait time of five years for a kidney. Organ procurement for deceased donor transplants contributes to 36% of the transplant cost. Considering these factors, the current estimated first-year cost for a deceased donor kidney is $216,000 compared to $138,000 for a living donor transplant.

A living donor kidney can typically be transplanted within a year of finding a qualified donor, reducing the need for repeated testing. Furthermore, kidneys from living donors last longer, meaning individuals with kidney failure would need fewer transplants over their lifetime. Living donor kidney transplants require fewer resources compared to hemodialysis, peritoneal dialysis, and deceased donor transplants.

The Bias Against Living Kidney Donation

It is essential to provide everyone with chronic kidney disease access to information about the best treatment option: living kidney transplantation. Early discussions about transplantation options, preferably before or during kidney disease Stage 4, allow more time to find a living donor and plan ahead before starting dialysis.

With kidney transplants often not being offered as the primary treatment option, the majority of individuals end up on dialysis. The image titled "Current Reality of Dialysis vs. Kidney Transplant" illustrates this current situation, showing that 69% of people are on dialysis while only 31% have received a kidney transplant.

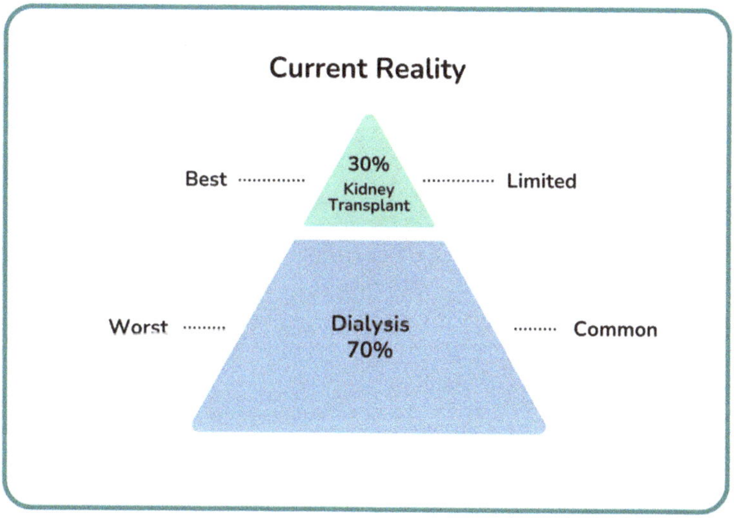

Current Reality of Dialysis vs. Kidney Transplant

As the duration of dialysis increases, overall health tends to decline, with only 15% of hemodialysis patients maintaining good physical condition after two years. Unfortunately, not everyone is initially healthy enough to qualify for a kidney transplant, and many individuals on dialysis may not receive sufficient guidance or education about the benefits of transplantation. It is crucial to discuss kidney transplant as early as possible, even if dialysis is the most suitable initial treatment for kidney failure. Ongoing discussions about transplantation should continue at regular intervals, as health conditions, social situations, attitudes, and understanding of consequences evolve over time.

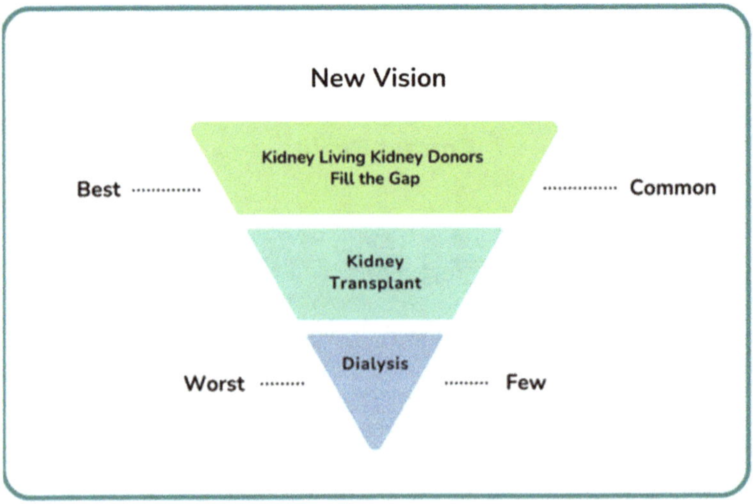

A New Vision for Kidney Transplants and Dialysis

The need for more living kidney donors is critical. Donating a kidney not only benefits the recipient but also helps reduce the deceased donor waitlist, enabling others to receive a transplant sooner. The image titled "A New Vision for Kidney Transplants and Dialysis" represents the hoped-for future for individuals with kidney failure.

There are significant barriers for living kidney donors. Currently, 65% of donors are female, 71% are white, 12% are Black, and 9% are Hispanic. These disparities stem from a range of cultural, social, economic, and personal factors. Not everyone has the resources needed to be a living kidney donor, such as paid time off work, travel funds, and coverage for other out-of-pocket expenses. While selling kidneys is illegal in the United States, there is ongoing discussion about ways to make donating easier by reducing disincentives and providing incentives. Ideally, no one should have to incur out-of-pocket expenses to donate a kidney.

Proposals to support living donors include:

- Reimbursement for travel and housing expenses related to testing, surgery, follow-up, and recovery
- Reimbursement for lost wages
- Reimbursement for adult care and child care
- Tax incentives
- Government compensation program for all donors
- Health and/or life insurance

One proposed solution to address the kidney shortage is to offer $45,000 through the U.S. government for kidney donation. This approach could potentially save thousands of lives each year and save taxpayers approximately $12 billion annually. The feasibility of this proposal is supported by the cost savings associated with preventing and reducing the need for dialysis and reducing the number of people on the transplant waiting list. Establishing a trial program with such incentives is considered a critical step forward.

The Coalition to Modify NOTA was established to address the shortcomings of the current system in handling the kidney failure crisis in the United States. The Coalition supports modifying the National Organ Transplant Act to allow government compensation for donors in a manner that is neither exploitative nor coercive. They propose the End Kidney Deaths Act, a ten-year pilot program offering a refundable tax credit of $10,000 per year for five years (totalling $50,000) to living kidney donors who donate to strangers. By the tenth year of the program, up to 100,000 Americans could receive healthy kidney transplants, potentially saving taxpayers up to $37 billion. In 1984, Representative Al Gore, a co-author of the Act, suggested that if efforts to improve voluntary donation failed, incentives such as tax credits should be considered. It is time to revisit this idea for supporting living kidney donors.

Insights for the Chapter: Treatment for Kidney Failure

- Kidneys are complex organs that filter our blood to help us stay healthy, and one healthy kidney cleans our blood better than dialysis.
- Living donor transplants last longer than deceased donor transplants and provide a cost savings compared to hemodialysis, peritoneal dialysis, and deceased donor transplants.
- More support is needed for living kidney donors so more lives can be saved.
- Watch this 15-minute YouTube video: **Understanding Living Kidney Donation** at https://youtu.be/ng8n6VXya1A?si=bZ-oCx0_PnKlGpCB

Champions keep playing until they get it right.

~Billie Jean King

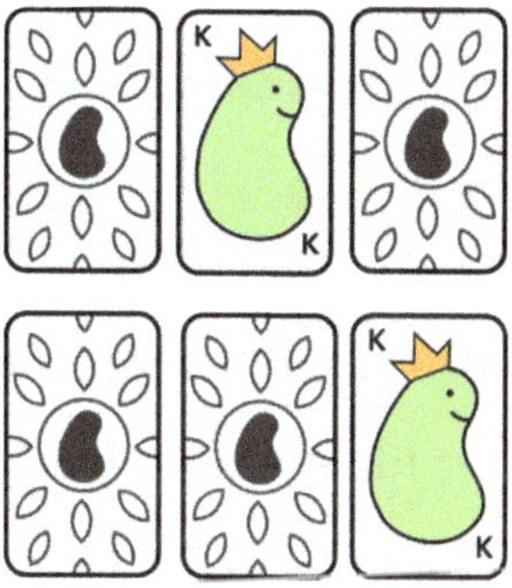

KIDNEY MATCHING

When people first consider donating or receiving a kidney, one important factor to consider is whether the donor and recipient are compatible or a match. Many people believe that being a match just means the same blood type, but there are other issues that are considered, such as:

- Blood type or ABO antigens
- Human leukocyte antigens (HLA)
- Crossmatch
- Size of the kidney
- Age of the donor and recipient

Most people want to donate to a specific person (referred to as their intended recipient) and are often told they are a "perfect match." Unfortunately, there is no standard definition for "perfect match" because the HLA tissue typing that is done is extremely complex, and different centers may have different ways of testing and reporting results. The match is likely "good enough" for the intended recipient. Something that may not be discussed is that another **even better matched recipient** could be found for the donor. And it is likely that an **even better matched donor** could be found for the original intended recipient. A closer match between donor and recipient leads to a longer-lasting kidney transplant. Using large kidney registries can provide access to a larger number of donors and recipients for better matching. Kidney registries are discussed later in this chapter.

A kidney transplant doesn't last forever because the body's immune system is at work. The body naturally fights against anything it thinks is foreign, like germs or viruses. This is how the immune system keeps people healthy. It attacks anything unfamiliar, thinking it might be harmful. When someone gets a new kidney from another person, their immune system doesn't know the kidney is helpful, so it attacks or "rejects" it.

Human leukocyte antigen (HLA) tissue typing is the method to match kidneys. This looks at genetic codes to find kidneys that are similar to those of the person who needs one. Identical twins have the same genes, so one twin can give a kidney to the other without problems. For everyone else, they try to find kidneys with close HLA matching, but this is complex and can be a challenge. When a kidney transplant is well-matched to the person receiving it, their body is less likely to see it as foreign or bad. This means the immune system won't attack the new kidney as much.

Even with HLA matching, people with a kidney transplant still need to take special medications called immunosuppressants. These drugs suppress or lessen the immune system. This makes it more difficult to fight something foreign in the body and decreases the chance of attacking the new kidney. Unfortunately, the body does not fight infections as well with these drugs, so it's easier to get sick. There can also be unwanted side effects, so it's best to use the lowest dose of drugs that can prevent the immune system from attacking the kidney.

Those who receive a kidney transplant have a slow, long-term development of antibodies that are fighting against the kidney. This antibody attack continues for the life of the kidney. That is why kidneys only last about 10–20 years. This happens even with the immunosuppressant drugs and even if a kidney is "a perfect match" or "compatible." Those terms do not correlate with how long the kidney will actually last.

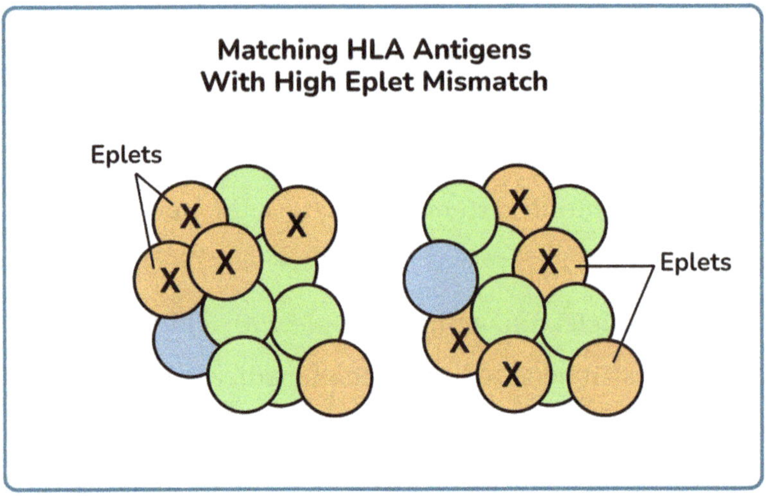

Technology has made a potentially better matching system called high-resolution tissue typing available. This high-resolution tissue typing looks at smaller parts of the HLA called eplets. When donor and recipient eplets are compared, some of them will be considered matched, and the rest of them are considered mismatched. The fewer that are *not* a match, the more likely the kidney is to last longer. Even if the HLA is "a good match" between donors and recipients, there could be high eplet mismatches within the HLA. As an example, the image titled "Matching HLA Antigens With High Eplet Mismatch" shows two HLA antigens that are the same. But when considering the eplet matching, they are a high eplet mismatch because four out of the five yellow eplets do not match.

Eplet matching may provide the following benefits:

- Increased likelihood of finding a more compatible kidney donor
- A lower risk of:
    - developing antibodies to attack the kidney
    - rejection episodes in the transplanted kidney
    - the transplanted kidney failing
- Lower doses of the immune-suppressing drugs
- Fewer side effects from the drugs

This high-resolution tissue typing using eplets is still new and has some challenges:

- Few clinical studies
- No long-term clinical studies
- Not all doctors and transplant centers use this method
- It costs more money than other ways of matching
- It takes longer to complete the test, so it cannot be used for deceased donor transplants
- There is not a public list of the transplant centers that provide this testing

Find out if transplant centers offer high-resolution eplet tissue typing. If this service is not provided, ask where it can be accessed. In addition, ask about the benefits eplet matching may provide for the donor and recipient. Children may benefit the most since they will likely need several transplants in their lifetime. Older recipients may not benefit as much since the kidney does not need to last as long compared to a younger recipient.

Some living kidney donors may be faced with an unexpected matching issue. If someone plans to donate to a family member, testing may reveal that the donor and recipient are not related. It can uncover that the person thought to be the father is **not** the biologic father and is called "misattributed paternity." This can create a difficult situation for donors and recipients if this is a new discovery for one or both of them. Transplant centers should have a policy and plan for how to handle these test results. Informing potential donors of this possibility in advance is important. Discussions should take place about whether or not donors want to be informed of the results, if this occurs.

Insights for the Chapter: Kidney Matching

- Kidney matching has historically been done using **HLA (human leukocyte antigens).**

- **High resolution eplet** matching may provide better matched kidneys that last longer than HLA matching.
- Watch this 3-½-minute YouTube video: **Why A Kidney Transplant Won't Last Forever** at https://youtu.be/EPocEXPTKQ4?si=1UrVOw1gSBgd0dS2

When faced with a decision,
choose the path that
feeds your soul.

~Dorothy Mendoza Row

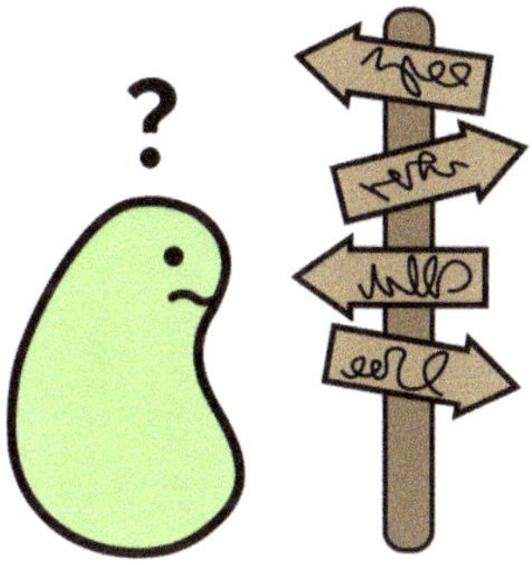

Ways to Donate a Kidney

It may be surprising to learn that there are different options, benefits, and protections, depending on how living kidney donors choose to donate. These can be different depending on the transplant center and which kidney registries they work with. For example, if a center does not offer a voucher donation option, the potential recipient or donor may never be told about voucher information. Another example is that a non-directed donation to a stranger may offer greater benefits than donating directly to a specific person.

The information below outlines the various options for living donors.

Ways to Donate a Kidney

Beyond deceased donation, there are three basic ways to be a living kidney donor. Each of these options will be examined in more detail.

1. Directed
2. Donor Exchange
    a. Paired Donation
    b. Chains
3. Non-Directed
    a. Voucher Donation

I have designed a pyramid image to illustrate the broad benefits of the different types of donation for recipients. (Refer to diagram "Kidney Donation Types.") Non-directed donation is listed on the top as the "best" because of the potential for starting a chain and helping the most number of people on the transplant waiting list.

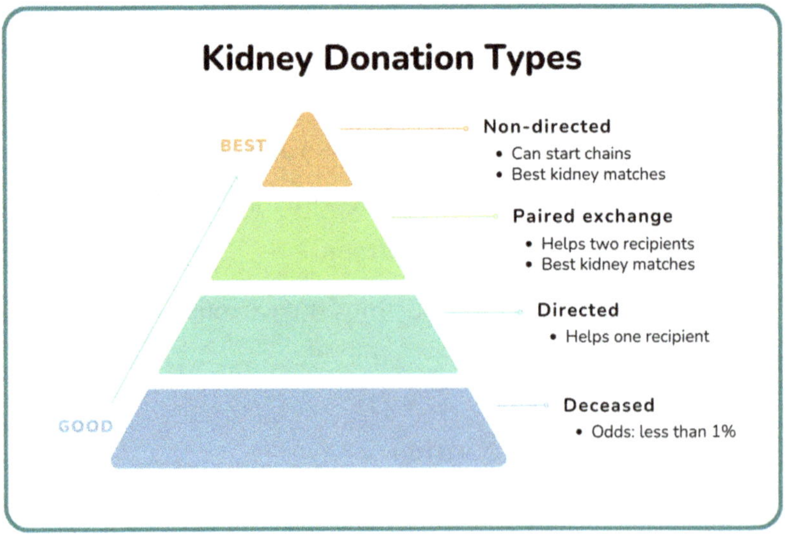

Directed Donation

If a family member, friend, or co-worker has kidney disease and needs a kidney transplant, it may be possible to give a kidney directly to them. This is a directed donation. The kidney is donated to a specific person. The donor may be related to the person, but does not need to be. The person who needs the kidney is called the intended recipient.

Testing is needed to ensure donors are healthy enough and are compatible with the intended recipient. Details of the screening and testing process can be found in the chapters discussing Stage 4 ("Initial Screening") and Stage 5 ("Full Workup").

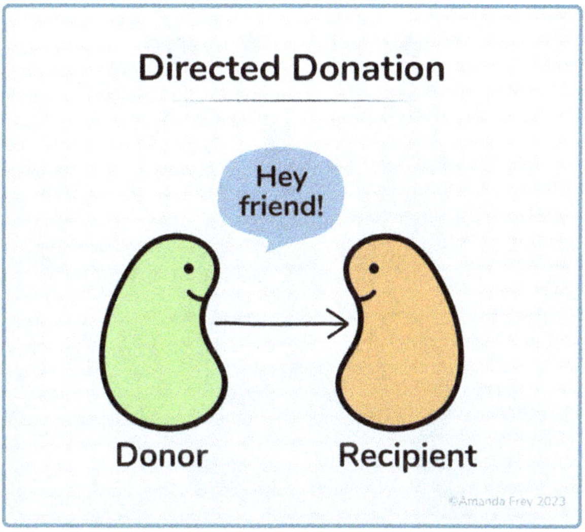

If a donor is healthy but does not match the intended recipient, they can still donate through a paired exchange or a non-directed donation. Unfortunately, many potential donors stop the donation process, not knowing there are other options.

Donor Exchange

When a potential donor does not have the correct blood type or is incompatible with the intended recipient, a kidney donor exchange can be an option.

One type of donor exchange is called a kidney swap, paired exchange, or paired donation.

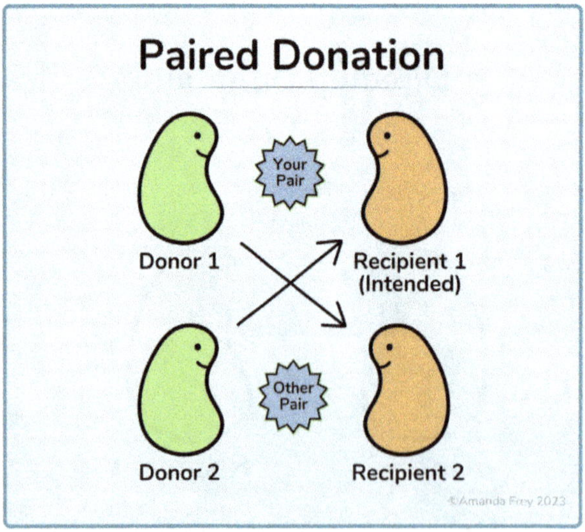

The donor and intended recipient are called a pair. There are other pairs like them, made up of people who need a kidney and those who want to donate to them, but they don't match each other. All of these pairs are put into a computer program called a registry. The program then finds people who are compatible. For example, Donor 1 is matched with Recipient 2, while Donor 2 is matched with Recipient 1. Often, better matched kidneys are found this way because many people are in the registries, waiting to be matched.

> *Even if donors and recipients are not compatible, they can participate in a paired donation, allowing the intended recipient to receive a kidney transplant.*

Kidney Chains

The second type of donor exchange is a chain. A kidney chain is a way to help many people get matching kidneys when their own loved ones can't give them one directly. Organizing a chain can be quite complex. The living donor and recipient transplant coordinators at the transplant centers collaborate closely with the transplant and surgery teams, often across different states. The process can take place over months or years and is worth helping so many people receive life-saving transplants. In the U.S., kidney chains provide kidneys to an average of more than four people.

Closed Kidney Chain

In a closed kidney chain, there are an equal number of donor and recipient pairs. The pairs go into a computer registry system to be matched. (Refer to image "Closed Chain.") In this example, Donor 1 is matched with Recipient 2. Donor 2 is matched with Recipient 3. And Donor 3 is matched with Recipient 1, which closes the chain.

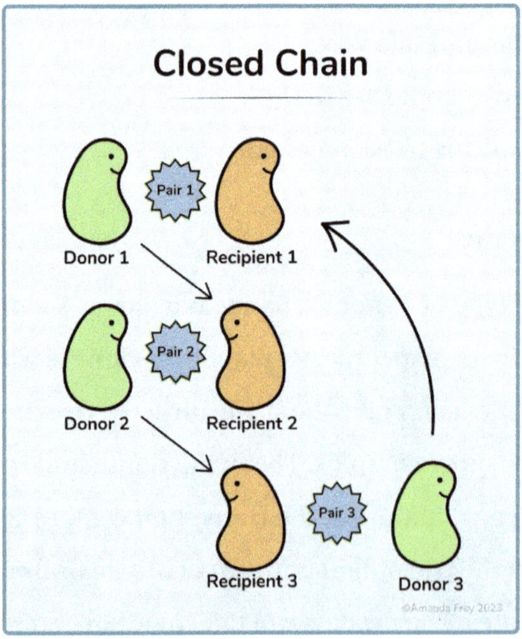

Open or Non-Directed Kidney Chain

An open or non-directed kidney chain is also called a daisy chain or a non-simultaneous extended altruistic donor chain (NEAD). It includes donor and recipient pairs who want to be matched, like in the closed kidney chain. The main difference is that **this chain is started by a non-directed donor.** Non-directed donors are willing to donate their kidney to a stranger, regardless of who the recipient is. The donor and recipient surgeries may take place the same day or can be separated by days, months, or years. (Refer to image "Non-Directed Chain.") In this example, Recipient 1 is not matched with anyone in the chain. Donor 1 will not give their kidney away until a kidney match is found for Recipient 1, so the chain cannot begin. Then, a non-directed Donor is matched with Recipient 1. Donor 1 is now willing to donate to Recipient 2 and the chain is started. It takes a non-directed living donor to start this chain.

Sometimes a donor in a chain does not have a recipient match when the other transplants are taking place. In this example, Donor 3 will be matched with a recipient at a later time and might start a chain in the future. This is called a bridge donor. They are like a bridge between two kidney chains.

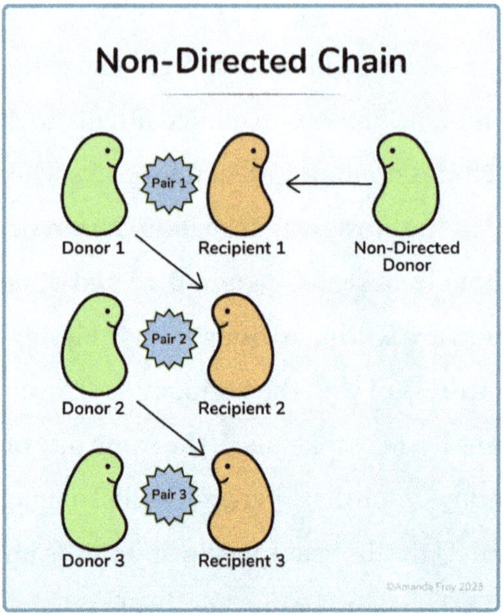

According to Guinness World Records, the longest kidney transplant chain was in 2015 and involved 35 transplants through the National Kidney Registry. It was started by a non-directed donor. The nation's longest ongoing single-site kidney chain occurred at the University of Alabama at Birmingham. There have been 126 transplants in this chain since 2023.

Non-Directed Donation

As mentioned in the section above about chains, there are some people who choose to donate their kidney to someone they do not personally know. This is called non-directed donation, donating to a stranger, altruistic donation, or a Good Samaritan donation.

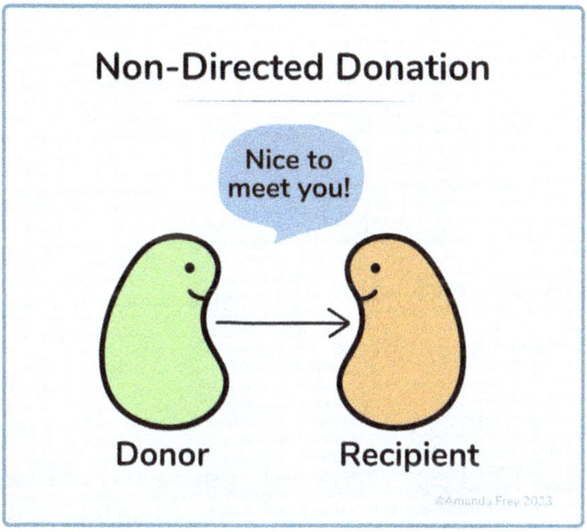

Sometimes, people are inspired to consider being a living kidney donor, even if they don't have a recipient in mind. They may learn about this option through news stories, social media, or movies. Some witness their loved ones die from kidney failure and want to prevent others from experiencing the same loss. The non-directed donor is entered into a registry to be matched with a compatible recipient. If their recipient is part of a pair in an exchange, the donor may be starting a kidney chain. Starting a chain can be the link that allows several families to experience the benefits of a transplant.

Support for Non-Directed Donors

Donors who give kidneys to strangers help society the most. They can start long chains of kidney donations, assisting many people waiting for transplants. More could be done to support those who want to donate a kidney. A few ideas include:

> *Non-directed kidney donors may start chains that can benefit the most number of people on the kidney transplant waiting list.*

- **Set up a single, government-funded list of living kidney donors (registry) that all transplant centers use.** This would allow for better matching opportunities because of a larger number of kidney donors to choose from. A better matched kidney means the transplant will likely last longer for the recipient and fewer transplants will be needed in their lifetime.
- Set up one easy government-funded voucher program for **kidney donors.** This program should not limit who can be designated to get a kidney in the future. Nor should it require anyone to anticipate when the kidney may be needed. Having many types of voucher systems is confusing for donors, recipients, families, and friends.

- **Require all transplant centers to participate in a single government-funded voucher program.** If more centers offered vouchers, it is likely that more people would come forward to be non-directed kidney donors. More non-directed donors would decrease the waiting time to get a transplant. More people would receive transplants. More lives would be saved.

Living Kidney Donor Registries and Benefits

Kidney registries are complex computer programs. Living kidney donor registries can be confusing to both the public and to most healthcare workers. Understanding the difference between the transplant waiting list for deceased donors and registries for living donors may be difficult. The **transplant waiting list** includes people with kidney disease who want a kidney from someone who has died, a deceased donor.

Living donor registries contain two lists. One list has people with kidney disease who want a kidney from a living donor. The other list has people who are approved to donate their kidney while alive through a paired exchange or as a non-directed donor. Registries were developed to compare these two lists and find the best matched living donor transplants for recipients. Many people are involved in managing the matching process and coordinating the details of living kidney donation and transplant.

There are many types of kidney registries, and this adds to the confusion about registries. Each transplant center may have its own internal system or registry for matching living donors and recipients. In addition, there are three major registries in the United States. Transplant centers may pay fees for membership to one or more registries. That means in total, there are likely over 250 registries (transplant centers and major registries) that are matching living donors and recipients.

Large Kidney Registries in the U.S.

Registry	Number of Transplant Centers *(January 2025)*
Alliance for Paired Kidney Donation (APKD)	45
National Kidney Registry (NKR)	103
United Network for Organ Sharing (UNOS) Kidney Paired Donation (KPD)	40

Donors and recipients may not know if a specific transplant center is aligned with a registry, and staff may not automatically share this during the workup process. Ask the coordinator if the transplant center participates in a kidney registry.

Besides the registry matching process, specific donor benefits may be available through a registry, particularly for non-directed donors. For instance, the National Kidney Registry offers the Donor Shield program, which provides extensive support and protections for donors. More details can be found at https://www.donor-shield.org/. The Alliance for Paired Kidney Donation offers a DonorProtect program, detailed at https://paireddonation.org/donorprotect/.

The National Living Donor Assistance Center (NLDAC) provides government grants for non-medical expenses for donors and is independent of registries and transplant centers. The income cutoff to receive funds is based on the recipient (not the donor). Non-directed donors can also apply, even though the recipient is not yet known. Applications may be submitted by paper or online once the donor workup process has begun, and they are finalized through the transplant center staff—typically the social worker. There is a proposal to amend the law so that funds are provided based on the donor, rather than the recipient income. Unfortunately, due to the income limit, many living donors do not qualify for the funds.

New York became the first state to reimburse costs associated with donating to living kidney and liver donors.

Governor Kathy Hochul signed the New York State Living Donors Support Act in 2023. Up to $10,000 may be provided for donation-related expenses, including lost wages, travel, lodging, childcare, medications, and medical care. Both the donor and recipient must be New York residents to qualify.

Some registries and transplant centers offer remote donation as a way to minimize out-of-pocket expenses. This allows donors to have surgery closer to home when donating to someone in a distant city, reducing travel and lodging costs for the workup process, transplant surgery, and follow-up care. Since donors may be advised not to fly for about a week after surgery, remote donation allows them to recover at home instead of in a hotel.

Voucher Donation

Two of the larger registries offer another option for living kidney donors called advanced or voucher donation. This allows a non-directed kidney donor to help someone immediately and also help someone who needs a kidney in the future. Few people are aware of advanced voucher programs, and many healthcare workers lack knowledge about these programs. If a transplant center does not offer a voucher option, this may never be discussed with potential kidney donors or recipients.

Many people are fearful of donating their kidney. One of the most common reasons for not wanting to donate their kidney is the fear that their children may need a kidney in the future. They don't want to take the chance of giving a kidney away today, when it may be needed later by their child. However, by the time the child is an adult and needing a transplant, the parent may no longer be a good candidate to be a donor.

Through a voucher program, a living donor is matched with a stranger in immediate need of a kidney. The donor receives a voucher (like a coupon) to give to a family member or friend, who can redeem it for a future kidney match if they progress to kidney failure. This process is like a paired donation separated in time. It is important to note that even if many people are listed on the voucher, only one person will be able to be matched with a kidney. (Refer to image "Voucher Donation") Recipient 1 does not currently need a kidney. Donor 1 provides a non-directed kidney donation to a stranger (Recipient 2) and names Recipient 1 on the voucher. Later, when Recipient 1 needs a kidney transplant, the voucher is turned in and they are placed into a registry and are matched with Donor 2.

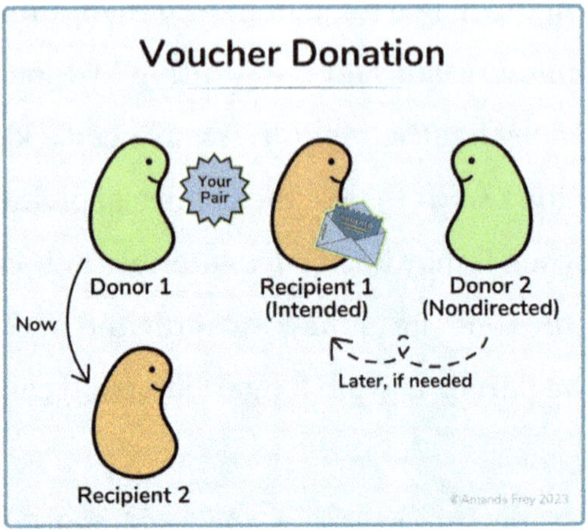

A broad way to look at vouchers is to categorize them as short term and long term. A **short-term voucher** is useful when someone with kidney disease is expected to need a kidney transplant within five years. Here are some examples:

- A 58-year-old man is the caregiver for his wife, who is on hemodialysis three times a week. He would like to donate his kidney to her but does not want to have surgery at the same time. He is matched with a stranger as a non-directed donor, providing his wife with a voucher. Once he's fully recovered from surgery, his wife can turn in the voucher to be matched with a kidney. Following her transplant surgery, he can now care for her.
- A 35-year-old school teacher prefers to donate her kidney in late June when school is not in session. This is not a good time for her friend, who won't be ready for a

kidney until a few months later because they are recovering from an infection. The school teacher is matched with a stranger as a non-directed donor, providing her friend with a voucher. When her friend is healthy enough to receive a transplant in October, they turn in the voucher to be matched with a kidney.

A **long-term voucher** is useful when a loved one is listed in the voucher but there is not an immediate need for a kidney. Here are some examples:

> *Because non-directed donors do not have a designated recipient, they may want to take more time exploring options and benefits available through different registries and transplant centers.*

- Children, family members, or friends who are currently healthy but may potentially require a kidney in the future, even if they are not at risk for kidney disease.
- Individuals with conditions like diabetes, high blood pressure, or polycystic kidney disease who currently have normal kidney function but may face kidney failure if their condition progresses.
- People who have already undergone a kidney transplant but may require a second or third transplant in the future. Kidney transplants typically last between 10 and 20 years, so this situation is especially important for

anyone who received their first transplant in their forties or younger.

Donating a kidney to a stranger now and obtaining a voucher for a loved one to use in the future could be a great solution in all of these situations. Often, donors can list more than one person in the voucher, even though only one person will be able to be matched with a kidney.

Voucher program information changes rapidly, and registries have several voucher options. The Alliance for Paired Kidney Donation voucher option is called Kidney Pledge. Details can be found at https://paireddonation.org/donorprotect/. The National Kidney Registry voucher programs can be found at www.kidneyregistry.org/for-donors/voucher-program.

A list of the transplant centers that participate in the National Kidney Registry can be found at www.KidneyTransplantCenters.org.

It is worth exploring the options and benefits available through registries and transplant centers before making a decision about the type of kidney donation, where to donate a kidney, or where to get a kidney transplant. Taking a proactive approach could provide a better understanding of available options and could potentially save significant costs.

Insights for the Chapter: Ways to Donate a Kidney

- The ways to donate a kidney include deceased, directed, donor exchange, and non-directed to a stranger.
- Registries play a critical role in the ways kidneys are matched, provide important benefits, and may offer a voucher donation option.
    - Watch this 8-½-minute YouTube video: **Living Kidney Donation Voucher Programs** at https://youtu.be/KIzTRLkmrIU
- Visit the **Kidney Donor Conversations** website at https://mykdc.org/learn-about-kidney-donation/, where information about transplant centers can be compared by selecting one of the following: "Click for Kidney Transplant Centers" and "Find the Best Hospital for You."

Nothing in life is to be feared, it is only to be understood.

~Marie Curie

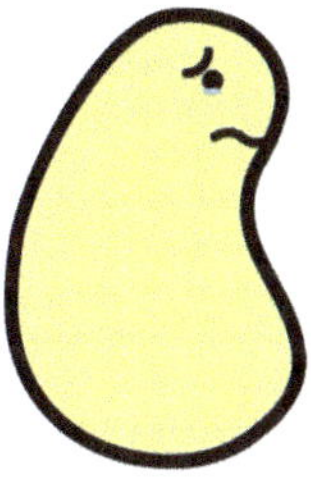

The Fear of Living Kidney Donation

Fear can influence people's decisions about living kidney donation. Fear is an emotional response to a perceived threat or danger, which can be real or imagined. It can be shaped by past experiences, cultural factors, and personality. Fear may exist at an unconscious level, and the causes of the fear may not be easily identified.

The information in this and the following chapters may help uncover specific fears about living kidney donation. These fears can be assessed by first identifying preferred donation methods. Then, step by step, facts about the living donation process may help to alleviate some of these fears.

Kidney Donation Continuum

Since founding the nonprofit Kidney Donor Conversations in 2018, we have had significant engagement with people about living kidney donation and have offered numerous educational presentations. Through these interactions, the Kidney Donation Continuum was developed, a simple scale that allows audience members to express their willingness to donate a kidney. This scale has been refined over time, and it takes just a minute to determine one's position on the continuum (refer to image "Kidney Donation Continuum").

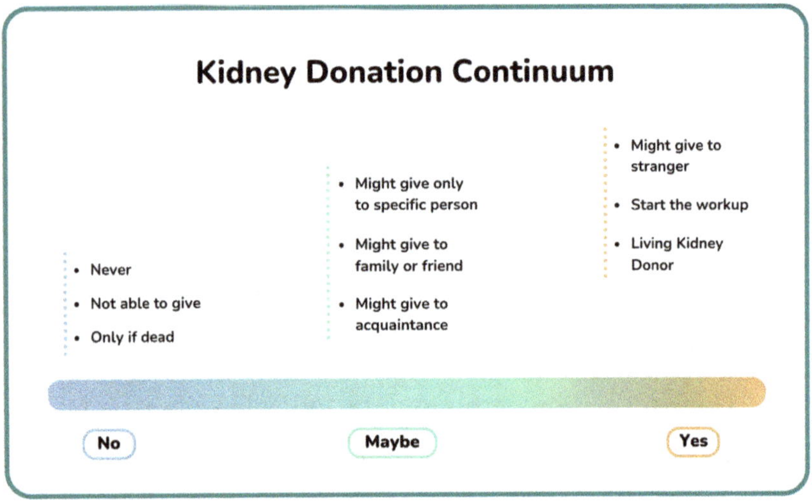

Many preferences emerge: some are willing to donate only to someone they know, while others are open to donating to anyone. Attitudes toward donation can change over time. Someone may not know anyone who needs a kidney now but may in the future, while others are ready to help a total stranger. The continuum helps individuals to consciously recognize and acknowledge their personal decisions about kidney donation, and positions on the continuum may shift over time.

When starting out as a young nurse in a hemodialysis unit, one might only consider donating their kidney to someone who would "take good care of it" and have no intention of donating. However, years later, they might be open to donating their kidney to a stranger. As individuals mature and develop a deeper comprehension of the lasting effects of kidney disease, this willingness may extend beyond saving the life of a loved one.

Overview of the Living Kidney Donor Stages

After delivering presentations about living kidney donation, listening to hundreds of other donors tell their stories, and donating a kidney myself, I have identified eight stages of the donation process. Transplant staff believe the process begins when someone wants to begin the health testing to donate. News headlines focus on the surgery, with pictures of donors and recipients hugging in hospital gowns afterward. But these are tiny moments in the journey. I developed the Living Kidney Donation Stages to provide an overview of the entire process, which starts earlier than most people imagine. (See image "Living Kidney Donation Stages.")

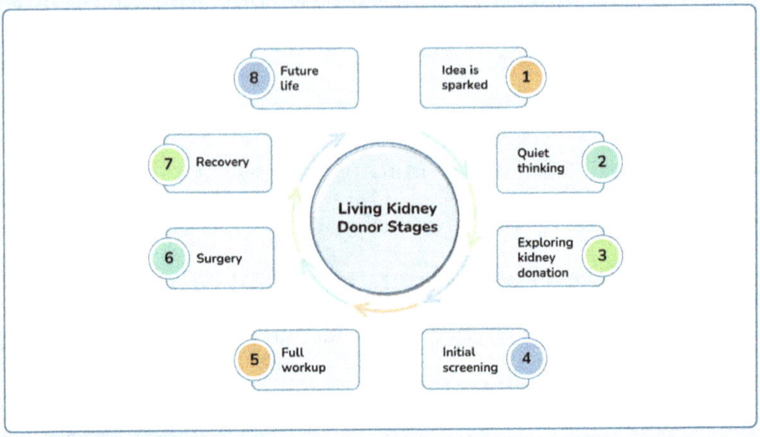

Healthcare professionals typically begin interacting with the potential donor at Stage 4: Initial Screening and may not acknowledge the first three stages. Donors may not go through the stages in the order listed. For example, exploring the details of donating may take place after the workup is started, rather than before. The length of each stage is different for each person based on motivation, physical health, mental health, family support, and work situations. Any one stage could go quickly or take years. The entire process could go quickly (less than one year) or slowly (many years). At any stage, the transplant center may determine the donor is not eligible to donate and the process stops.

No one should ever feel pressured into donating their kidney. As one moves forward, they are never locked into the decision to donate. At any point, the donation can be stopped and will be supported by the transplant team. Some fear is normal, but fear should not override the desire to donate. If the fear and anxiety of donating is still strong after gathering the facts and understanding the benefits and risks, then kidney donation may not be a good choice for that individual.

Peeking inside the process can offer a clearer and deeper understanding of this unique effort to help others. The hope is that reviewing these stages might reduce undue fear or anxiety, inspire greater curiosity about donation, and begin the process. The goal is always to minimize risk to the donor and optimize the chance of providing the recipient with a healthy, long-lasting kidney. However, there are no guarantees. The following chapters broadly describe each stage, even though every individual situation will be unique.

Insights for the Chapter:

The Fear of Living Kidney Donation

- The **Kidney Donation Continuum** may reveal hidden fears.
- The **Stages of Living Kidney Donation** provide a broad overview of the donation process; each person will have a unique, varied experience.

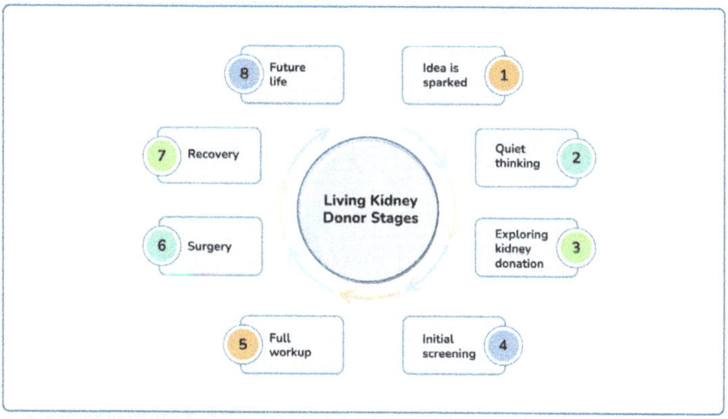

THE 8 LIVING KIDNEY DONATION STAGES

Tell me, what is it you plan to do with your one wild and precious life?

~Mary Oliver

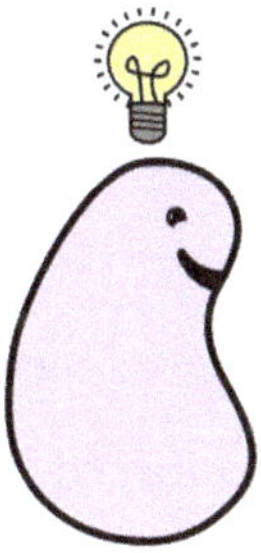

Stage 1: The Idea Is Sparked

Many believe the kidney donation process starts with the call to a transplant center. However, it actually begins two stages earlier, with the initial spark of the idea. The decision to donate a kidney often begins with hearing someone else's donation story, whether through a news story, social media post, television show, TED talk, podcast, or personal encounter.

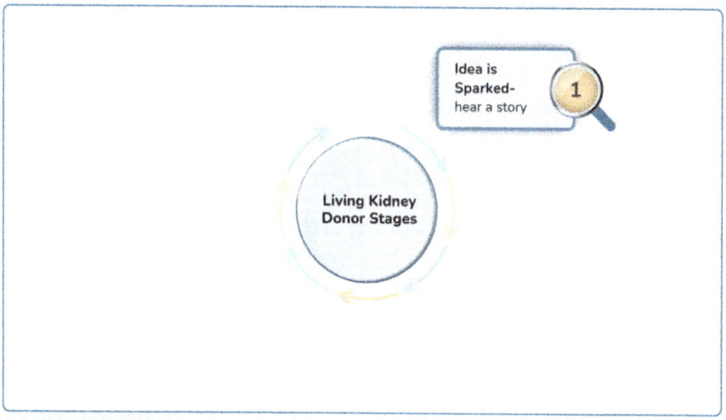

Or, people with kidney disease may be sharing their story of needing a kidney transplant. This can happen through various channels such as family, friends, co-workers, faith groups, hairdressers, teachers, or even strangers, with the permission of the person seeking a kidney. These stories often depict the challenges of life on dialysis, including physical hardships, reduced energy levels, difficulty working, and the battle to survive day to day. A kidney transplant has the potential to greatly improve their quality of life.

Planning to donate a kidney before the need for dialysis arises can help them live longer. For most people, life with a kidney transplant is superior to life on dialysis. Learning about someone who was near death, then regained vitality, energy, and function after a transplant can be deeply inspiring. Becoming a living kidney donor has the potential to save a life.

These stories may be the initial spark for someone to think about living donation. Some may experience thoughts like "I could do that" or "That could be me" or feel a chill down their spine upon hearing these stories. However, at Stage 1 of the Living Kidney Donor Stages, they are not yet prepared to voice the idea of potential donation. They are internally processing the information.

Insights for the Chapter: The Idea Is Sparked

- The spark is ignited by stories about other kidney donors or stories of someone needing a kidney transplant.

Don't focus on what
you can't do,
Focus on what you
can do.

~Glenna Frey

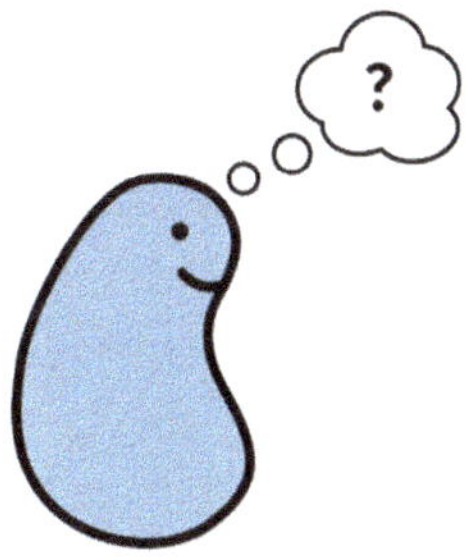

Stage 2: Quiet Thinking

Someone's silence on the matter of living kidney donation doesn't mean they aren't considering the idea of donating. Often, time is spent in quiet reflection before engaging with others about the topic. After hearing a story about someone who is in need of a kidney transplant or someone who has donated a kidney, the story continues to resonate in their thoughts. They ponder how one kidney can save the life of someone, especially those on dialysis.

Similar to Stage 1: The Idea Is Sparked, this stage may not be recognized by the healthcare team. Potential donors have not yet reached out to a transplant center. Because the idea of kidney donation is often feared and misunderstood, the thought of it can be overwhelming and not discussed. It may be difficult to consider donating to a stranger or narrowing the donation down to a specific known person who has kidney disease.

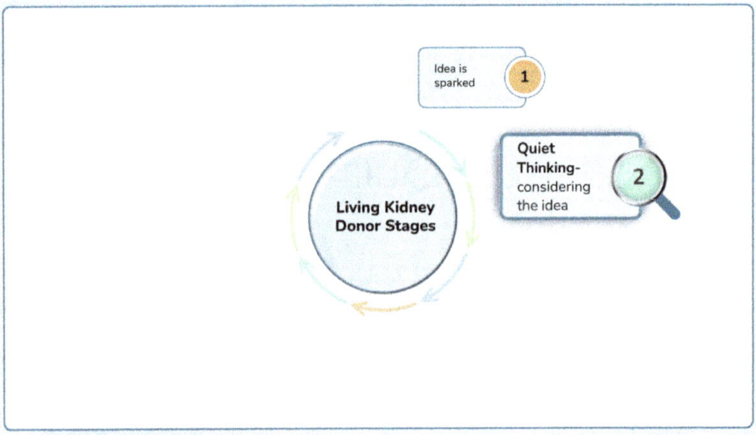

The idea of donating a kidney can be overshadowed by other concerns and life events. It may take time to process the thought of an elective surgery and its impact on family, friends, work, and life in general. At this early stage, there often isn't enough information about living kidney donation to make an informed decision. If there is any indication that friends and family may be critical, unsupportive, or unaware of the facts, it may feel easier to remain silent and contemplate the idea of donating alone.

Here are some examples of topics that potential donors may silently worry about before they have more facts or are willing to discuss these concerns with others:

- The fear of dying during surgery.
- How the surgery and recovery time will affect their family life, such as caregiving needs for young children or elderly parents. Additionally, planned weddings, vacations, or other important life events could be impacted by a major surgery.
- Donating directly to a family member such as a parent, spouse, or child means both surgeries would occur on the same day. As a result, both donor and recipient would be recovering from surgery at the same time, which could present more challenges.
- Uncertainty about whether living donation aligns with religious beliefs. If this topic hasn't been previously addressed, there could be hesitation to bring it up for fear of criticism or guilt.
- Uncertainty about how donating will affect their job, leading them to avoid informing co-workers or employers. They might lack the benefits or resources to take paid time off for the workup, surgery, and recovery. Additionally, they may not have the finances

to afford many weeks off without a steady income and to cover out-of-pocket donor expenses.

- They may avoid talking about donating until they are certain it is the right decision for them. Such discussions could bring unwanted attention and drama. Although they may like the idea of donating, it may not be the right time, they may not understand the process, or they may not have a specific recipient in mind.

All of these issues can be quite stressful to consider. As the possibility of donating continues to arise, it may take a long time to mentally process these concerns. During this stage, they may notice a persistent, gentle whisper, as though the universe is quietly calling them to help. The decision to move forward in this journey depends on many personal factors. When they are ready to learn more about the benefits and risks of donating, they are moving into Stage 3: Exploring Kidney Donation. This next stage may provide more clarity for donors.

Insights for the Chapter: Quiet Thinking

- Many fears may arise when considering the idea of donating a kidney.
- Silently reflecting on the idea of kidney donation is often necessary before discussing it with family or friends.

Everything's a risk.
Not doing anything
is a risk.
It's up to you.

~Nicola Yoon

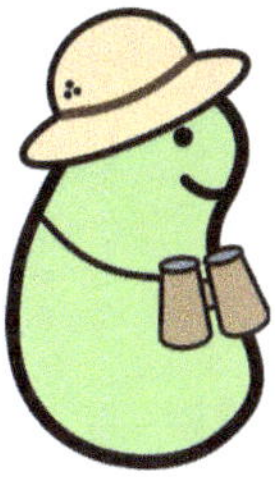

Stage 3: Exploring Kidney Donation (Criteria, Benefits, & Cost)

Often potential donors want to do something meaningful with their lives and make a special impact on others. However, they are fearful of the unknown and concerned about how donation might affect their future health. This chapter covers important facts for donors and families, including eligibility criteria, benefits, and costs.

This stage is unique because researching information about living kidney donation may take place before, after, or anywhere within the donation process. It expands throughout the process, intertwining with all the stages. As potential donors wonder if they can donate, they will not know for sure if donating is right for them until the workup is complete and surgery takes place. The following information may be helpful to consider.

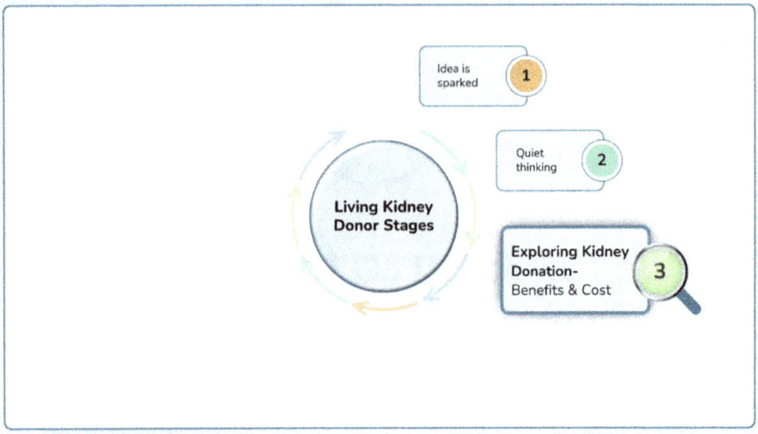

General Donation Criteria

The Organ Procurement and Transplantation Network (OPTN) is the regulating body that determines the minimum criteria for living kidney donors. Each transplant center also has their own policies that provide additional restrictions beyond what is regulated. Donors can be rejected at one center and be accepted at another. Some centers may require potential donors to make health modifications to meet the requirements, such as starting blood pressure medications or losing weight. It is not possible to compare policies across centers to make a more informed choice regarding which center may be optimal for the donor. The OPTN policy states: "Living donor recovery hospital may exclude a donor with any condition that, in the hospital's medical judgment, causes the donor to be unsuitable for organ donation." This can include medical or psychological conditions, such as doubts about the donor's motivation or concerns that they may be coerced into donating. For a potential donor, this can be a confusing and frustrating gray area. Many people exclude themselves as donors because they are not fully aware of the criteria and allowances at different transplant centers.

Providing a general idea of who would make a good living kidney donor candidate based on the OPTN policy is not possible. However, it is possible to share the exclusion criteria, which are reasons one cannot donate. Transplant centers may still deny donors for other reasons.

Donor age

Typically, living kidney donors are between 18 and 65, although there is no specific age limit. Legally, they must be at least 18. Being physically and mentally healthy with two healthy kidneys and good kidney function is a better measure than age. However, different transplant centers can have different policies. Some centers require donors to be **older** than 18, and there could be an **upper age limit**. The oldest living kidney donor in the United States is Frank Dewhurst, who donated in 2019 at the age of 84. Donors must also be deemed mentally capable of making informed decisions.

Donor Weight

The OPTN policy does not address weight, so weight cutoff is determined by each transplant center. Most often, body mass index (BMI) is the general unit of measure, using height and weight. BMI charts can easily be found online. Most transplant centers have a cutoff of 30, 35, or 40 BMI. Some donors who fall outside the center criteria are able to lose weight, then donate. It is interesting to note that most living kidney donors are in the overweight or obese categories yet are still allowed to donate. More research needs to be done on the long-term outcomes of donors in all weight categories. Weight loss, smoking cessation, and emotional support resources are available through Project Donor, a free program from the University of Chicago. This nonprofit organization helps organ donors meet donation criteria. More information can be found at https://projectdonor.org/.

Living Kidney Donor Exclusion Criteria

Here is a list of the other OPTN exclusion criteria.

Living Kidney Donor Exclusion Criteria

HIV	Unless certain criteria are met as outlined in Policy 15.7. A recipient must be willing to take an HIV positive donor.
Active Cancer	Cancer that is not fully treated, requires treatment, or has a risk of transmission.
Suspicion of inducement	Includes bribing, coercion, or undue pressure on a donor.
Suspicion of illegal exchange	Providing anything of value in exchange for the organ.
Active infection	Any active infection at the time of donation.
Uncontrolled Psychiatric Conditions	Including suicide risk.
Uncontrolled High Blood Pressure	Or high blood pressure with organ damage.
Diabetes	Type 1 or Type 2 with either organ damage or risk of complications.

Potential Living Kidney Donor Candidates

Here are some examples of health concerns and treatment that may still allow people to be a living kidney donor candidate.

Potential Living Kidney Donor Candidates

Blood Pressure	Controlled with one or two medications
Mental Health	Anti-anxiety and/or anti-depression medications are prescribed.
Cancer History	A history of certain cancers.
Weight	Overweight or obese.
Type 2 Diabetes	Diabetes is controlled with medications and/or diet.
HIV	May be able to donate to another person with HIV.

There are many differences between the various transplant centers. There is not currently a published comparison table that provides living donor selection criteria at each center. This can be frustrating for donors if they go to a center and are refused, but then go to another center and are accepted.

Selecting a Transplant Center

Here are factors to consider when selecting a transplant center. Asking about these issues early in the process can be beneficial. It's essential to choose the center that best meets personal needs.

- Directed donors may be asked to donate at the center where their intended recipient is registered. Planning ahead as early in the process as possible and exploring all options is crucial. Although challenging, discussing the option for the recipient to change centers may also increase their chances of receiving a living donor transplant.
- Location of the surgery may be determined by the recipient's insurance, which can involve complex issues. If the surgery location does not appear to be in the best interest of both the donor and recipient, there is a process to request an alternative arrangement. An appeal may be granted if there is strong rationale for selecting a different transplant center that offers better options. Donors and recipients can reach out to the financial adviser at the transplant center for necessary details and support. Recipients may also

> *Transplant centers have different health criteria.*
>
> *Donors may choose to go to another center if they are not accepted at the first one and still feel they could be a good candidate.*

wish to contact their insurance company with any questions or concerns.

- If the donor and recipient reside in different locations or states, the donor may feel pressured to have surgery at the recipient's transplant center, which could require more travel time and money. Some centers offer remote donation. With a remote donation, the donor has surgery at a conveniently located transplant center and the kidney is transported to a different center where the recipient will have surgery. Additional work may be necessary to explore and advocate for the option of remote donation before making a decision about the transplant center. This may be more difficult for directed donors and easier for non-directed donors.
- Donors may prefer a center with optimal patient and kidney survival rates, donor protections, donor benefits, or a voucher option. Information about kidney registries and related benefits can be found in the chapter "Ways to Donate a Kidney."
- If the donor cannot donate to their intended recipient, they might consider entering a donor exchange program, becoming a non-directed donor, or participating as a voucher donor (refer to Chapter 4: Ways to Donate a Kidney). Both the donor and recipient may need to make compromises to facilitate

the donation process. Effective communication is essential.

These websites offer information about transplant centers and can be useful.

Best Hospitals in Nephrology

Top Kidney Transplant Centers

Scientific Registry of Transplant Recipients (SRTR)

Donor Health

Potential donors undergo a thorough screening process to assess their current health, ensuring that any potential risks associated with donation are minimized. This testing is covered by the recipient's insurance and incurs no cost to the donor. Occasionally, this screening process reveals previously unknown medical issues, such as high blood pressure, diabetes, kidney disease, or cancer. Even if donation is not feasible, identifying these conditions early allows time for interventions, providing unexpected benefits. It is important to point out that routine health screening tests may be expected to be covered by the donor's insurance. (Refer to the chapter "Full Workup.")

Donating a kidney carries certain general health risks. As with any major surgery, there is a minor risk of death. This risk typically depends on factors such as the donor's health, internal anatomy, the surgeon's skill, and the coordination of the healthcare team.

Here are some of the risks specific to kidney donors and the chances of that risk occurring:

- The risk of death due to removing a kidney is 0.01%. This risk is lower than that of childbirth or gallbladder surgery.
- The risk of having a major complication within 90 days of surgery is 2.9%.
- The annual mortality risk of kidney donation is comparable to that of riding a bike, estimated at about 1 in 3,000. This risk is lower than the annual risk many face of dying in a car accident, which is about 1 in 100.

> *Living kidney donors live longer than the general population, not because they donated, but because they are healthier.*

- The average lifetime risk of kidney failure requiring dialysis or a transplant is 0.9% for kidney donors and 3.2% for the general population. Kidney donors are less likely to develop kidney failure not because their kidney was removed, but because they are generally healthier. Only the healthiest individuals are allowed to donate kidneys. If they develop kidney failure later in life, they will receive priority points to move higher up on the deceased donor transplant list.

- The risk of high blood pressure or preeclampsia during pregnancy is slightly higher in donors (11%) than non-donors (5%). It is important to be closely monitored during pregnancy. It is often recommended that pregnancy be delayed at least a year after donating.
- People of African ancestry may possess the APOL1 gene, which may increase the risk of kidney disease. It's important to discuss genetic testing options with living kidney donors who may be at risk. If testing is completed and the gene is identified, the potential donor and healthcare team should collaborate to decide whether to proceed with donation.
- Living kidney donors will have an average of 25–35% permanent loss of kidney function after donating. The remaining kidney works to compensate for the missing one to keep the body healthy. This is considered a normal response to donating and should not be assumed to be kidney disease.

Because statistics are general and not specific to individuals, risk calculators have been developed to help people determine their personal risk for donating a kidney.

By entering personal data into the calculators, one can estimate their risk compared to individuals with two kidneys who have similar data. Some information may need to be obtained from a healthcare provider, who can also explain the terminology and answer any medical questions, as some details in the calculators may be confusing. It is unclear how accurate the calculators are since there are not many long-term studies available on living kidney donors. (Refer to Appendix 2: Living Kidney Donor Risk Tools.)

Despite extensive screening, unanticipated problems or future issues related to kidney donation may still occur. Transplant centers aim to ensure that risks are minimal, both short-term and long-term, before removing a kidney. If the donor's risk is deemed too high, they will not be cleared to donate. This can be disappointing for individuals, but it is done for their safety. Many people who cannot donate become advocates for living donation or support those on the transplant waiting list. There are many ways to provide other types of support, such as:

- Spreading awareness about living donation
- Providing donors with meals, childcare, or transportation
- Supporting a kidney-related nonprofit

- Participating in a walk or fundraiser for donors or recipients

Donor's Time

Donating a kidney requires a time commitment, much like any other chosen endeavor. Each stage of the living kidney donation process involves dedicated time:

1. Full Workup: This stage typically involves travel time, extensive testing at the transplant center, and waiting for results. Sometimes further testing may be needed. Many donors report feeling frustrated due to the process not moving as quickly as hoped.
2. Preparation and Surgery: After completing the workup, there may be a wait for the surgery. Time is also needed for the pre-operative visit to prepare for surgery itself, followed by the procedure and recovery period in the hospital.
3. Recovery and Follow-Up: Recovery continues at home post-donation, followed by around four more follow-up visits back to the transplant center. Most transplant centers will follow donors for two years, with visits shortly post-donation, at six months, one year, and two years.

4. Long-Term Discussions: Even after donation, there may be ongoing discussions about the kidney donor experience, potentially lasting a lifetime.

Psychological Considerations

Along with the time commitment, the mental and emotional costs of kidney donation can come as a surprise to donors. It's beneficial to have support from family and friends throughout the process. Professional counseling is often overlooked and can be invaluable before, during, and after donation. Donors may experience stress related to concerns about the recipient's care of the transplanted kidney. Emotional highs and lows can persist for years. As donors age, these emotions may be influenced by changes in the donated kidney's function, the recipient's health, and the donor's own kidney function and health.

Hidden Donor Costs

The recipient's insurance pays for the cost of the donor workup and surgery, but there can be other costs associated with the donation process. The cost of donating a kidney can be measured in many ways. It could be actual dollars spent for travel, time off work for the workup, surgery, and recovery, as well as the physical and emotional energy that is expended.

The cost for donors varies depending on the donor's employer, time needed off work, family situation, distance from the transplant center, and time needed for recovery. Workplace benefits can vary. A discussion with a member of the company's human resources department can help a donor understand the benefits and considerations for time off.

Here is a list of some common costs:

- Travel (gas, car, bus, plane, etc.)
- Hotel & food
- Salary lost for time off work
- Cost for childcare or adult care if donor is a caregiver
- Pet sitting

For most, not only does the donor have costs, but close family and friends are also affected. Some transplant centers mandate that the donor have a caregiver present during the workup and for surgery. These support people may also need to take time off work, and may have travel expenses and other non-medical expenses similar to the donor's. Some registries and transplant centers may provide assistance with these expenses (refer to Chapter 4, "Living Kidney Donor Registries and Benefits"). It's crucial to recognize these hidden costs, as many donors and families may not initially consider them.

Itemizing the donor and support individual's costs in advance can better prepare everyone for these expenses. The American Society of Transplantation has developed a **Living Donor Toolkit: Resources for Those Considering Live Donation** that includes a **Living Organ Donation Cost-Estimation Worksheet.** This can be found at https://www.myast.org/sites/default/files/AST-16-Financial-Toolkit-Section-1-Cost-Estimation-Worksheet.pdf.

Several avenues exist to provide financial support for living kidney donors that may help with the non-medical expenses:

- The recipient may reimburse their donor for expenses, although most recipients may not be aware of this option or have the funds to do so.

> *On average, expenses (that do not include workup or surgery) for a living donor are over $1000 and as high as $10,000.*

- Some transplant centers, kidney registries, and organizations like Renewal (www.renewal.org) provide benefits for donors. Examples of benefits include:
    - Lost wage reimbursement
    - Travel and dependent care assistance

    - Legal support
- Other ways to be reimbursed for expenses include:
    - Personal fundraising
    - Applying for grant funding through the National Living Donor Assistance Center (NLDAC)
    - State benefits

The National Living Donor Assistance Center (NLDAC) is a federally funded program designed to assist eligible donors with travel, lost wages, and dependent care expenses. Potential donors should initiate the application process once their workup has begun. This typically starts with a discussion with the donor's social worker, who will then make the referral to NLDAC. Funding eligibility is based on the recipient's income, not the donor's. Non-directed donors can also apply, even though the recipient is not yet known at the time of the application. It's important to note that applications must be approved and funded before donation surgery.

Some states have living donor benefits. To find out more about state laws impacting organ donation, go to https://www.kidney.org/sites/default/files/ld_tax_ded_leave_20220603.pdf.

Religious Issues

Major religious organizations hold varying but generally supportive views on organ donation. Donation is typically supported as an act of compassion and potentially saving lives.

- Christianity: an act of love and helping others.
- Islam: allows under specific conditions, considering it a charitable act to save lives.
- Judaism: a mitzvah (commandment) to save lives, with guidelines for ethical consent.
- Hinduism: an act of compassion and good karma.
- Buddhism: positive, aligns with principles of compassion and reducing suffering.

For detailed religious views, consult official statements or scholars from each tradition, since interpretations can evolve over time.

Benefits of Kidney Donation

The testing to determine the health of a potential donor is covered by the recipient's insurance. Therefore, donors get a thorough physical and psychosocial workup at no charge. This process may uncover previously unknown medical conditions such as high blood pressure, kidney disease, or cancer, offering early intervention and improved outcomes. Regardless of the ability to donate, this health information can be valuable. Many potential donors feel disappointed if unable to donate, while others may feel relief. Counseling can be beneficial for helping to process these feelings and emotions.

Donors understand the profound impact of improving a recipient's quality of life, especially if they have a close relationship. Transitioning from the draining routine of dialysis to seeing the recipient regain energy and function at a higher level can be incredibly rewarding.

Other benefits include:

- Increased self-esteem.
- High long-term health-related quality of life.
- Higher positive mental health than the general population.
- Because donors are so healthy at the time of donation, they tend to keep up that healthy lifestyle after donating.
- Improved relationship with recipient (for example: a new friend, closer relationship, reduced caregiver burden, financial benefits, or a return to normalcy).
- They would donate again if they could.

Experiencing the living donation process, whether for a stranger or someone close, evokes a deep sense of pride and satisfaction. This unique feeling is not always easy to explain. Nothing quite compares to voluntarily going through an unnecessary surgery, donating an organ, and helping to save a life.

Stage 3: Exploration can span from a matter of hours to many years before a potential donor reaches out to a transplant center. Additional information continues to be gathered throughout the donation process and beyond. Many donors discuss living kidney donation during this stage and those that follow, aiming to increase awareness and educate others.

Insights for the Chapter: Exploring Kidney Donation

- Potential donors should understand the transplant center criteria regarding age, BMI, cancer, infections, blood pressure, and diabetes before self-excluding.
- Conversations about the selection criteria, time commitment, associated costs, and benefits of donating help foster understanding and break the silence and mystery surrounding living donation.
- Refer to Appendix 3: Living Kidney Donation Resources for a list of organizations, books, Facebook pages, and podcasts that may be helpful while exploring living kidney donation.

Challenges make you discover things about yourself that you never really knew.

~Cicely Tyson

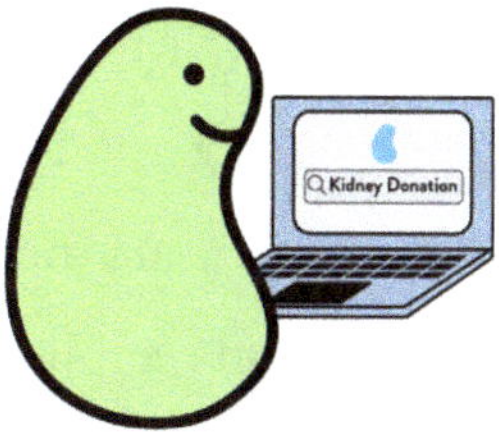

Stage 4: Initial Screening

For those considering kidney donation and wondering if they're healthy enough to proceed, an initial screening can be done privately at home.

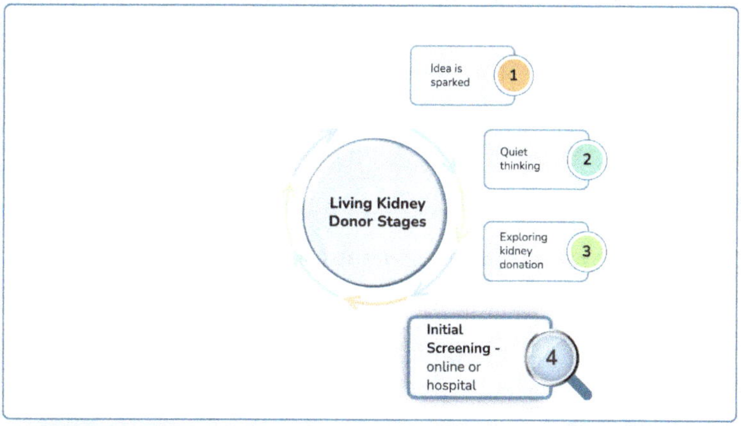

This step can help determine general health status before committing to donate or discussing it with others. Here are options for the online health questionnaire:

1. National Kidney Registry (NKR): Visit the homepage of the NKR at www.kidneyregistry.org. The initial screening information provided will start the process. You do not need to know the potential recipient or transplant center, and there is no commitment to donate through an NKR hospital to begin.
2. National Kidney Donation Organization (NKDO): Go to https://www.nkdo.org/considering-kidney-donation/. There is a direct link to the National Kidney Registry health questions for potential donors to start the initial screening.
3. Kidney Donor Conversations (KDC): Go to www.MyKDC.org. There is a direct link on the homepage to the National Kidney Registry health questions, making it easy for potential donors to start the initial screening.

After the initial health questionnaire is completed and approved, supplies for urine and blood samples can be sent for collection through a local lab. The bloodwork provides a reflection of the general physical health of your body and organs. If the results are within normal ranges, emails will be sent with guidance for the next steps.

The National Kidney Registry (NKR) has partnered with the National Kidney Foundation and the National Kidney Donation Organization to offer support phone calls with a living kidney donor for individuals using the NKR website.

The support aims to provide valuable information and assistance throughout the donation process.

The thorough in-person workup required for living kidney donation can only be done through a transplant center. To assist in choosing a center, the National Kidney Registry provides a link to compare U.S. transplant center services at https://www.kidneytransplantcenters.org/.

4. Most transplant centers have a link to donor intake questions on their website. A transplant center can be selected based on transplant center data, proximity, or the location where the intended recipient is going, depending on individual circumstances and preferences.

   The answers to these questions may help guide the choice of a transplant center. This center is typically where testing and the surgery will be done, although the recipient's location may influence the decision:

   - Is there an identified recipient?
   - Is there a state, city, or hospital that is preferred?
   - Is there a preference for a large transplant center or a small one?
   - Is traveling several hours or across the country an option?
   - If a remote donation is needed, can the kidney travel, instead of the donor?

- Is the transplant center near family or friends who can provide support and aid in recovery?
- What type of donor benefits are available at the transplant center that may be important? (e.g., low-cost accommodations, participation in the National Kidney Registry voucher program or the Alliance for Paired Kidney Donation KidneyPledge, lost wage reimbursement, travel and lodging reimbursement, etc.)
- What is the reputation and success rate of surgeries at the transplant center?
- Helpful websites:
  - Best Hospitals in Nephrology
  - Top Kidney Transplant Centers

Organizations that may provide additional guidance:

- Donor Outreach for Veterans (DOVE): A nonprofit organization aimed at improving access to living kidney transplants for veterans. DOVE provides education, screening, and support to potential donors and matches them to a veteran on the kidney transplant waiting list. Kidney transplants are performed through the Veterans Administration National Transplant Program. More information can be found at https://www.dovetransplant.org/new-donor and www.va.gov/health/services/transplant/.

- Renewal: A nonprofit organization based in New York that has streamlined the process of living kidney donation by working with transplant centers. More information is available at www.renewal.org.

Once a potential donor initiates contact with a transplant center, they will be connected with an Independent Living Donor Advocate. Transplant programs are required to provide this advocate to ensure the protection of donor rights. Donors have an interview with the Independent Living Donor Advocate before the donor evaluation begins. This advocate is not part of the transplant center donor evaluation team or the recipient's transplant team and is focused solely on the best interests of the potential donor.

Insights for the Chapter: Initial Screening

- The first easy step toward discovering if someone can be a living donor can be done at home with an online health questionnaire.
- Personal preferences and values can guide the selection of a transplant center after considering recipient needs and detailed transplant center information, including benefits for the donor.

You gain strength, courage, and confidence by every experience in which you really stop to look fear in the face. You must do the thing you think you cannot do.

~Eleanor Roosevelt

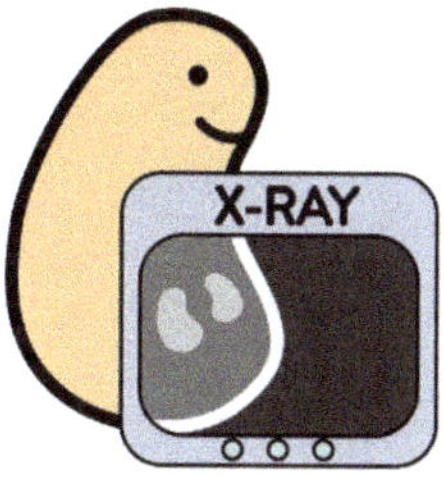

Stage 5: Full Workup

Potential donors are often surprised at the complexity of the testing required for the full workup. This process usually takes at least two full days and includes multiple tests, as well as interviews and education sessions with various healthcare team members. Living organ donation is the most highly regulated surgery, with specific requirements set by the Organ Procurement and Transplantation Network (OPTN) and the Centers for Medicare and Medicaid Services (CMS) regulations. It is interesting to note that while OPTN policies apply to all transplant programs, the CMS Conditions of Participation only apply to programs seeking Medicare payment for transplant services, excluding Veterans Affairs transplant centers. Additionally, each transplant center has its own policies, which may include more specific criteria and varying workup requirements.

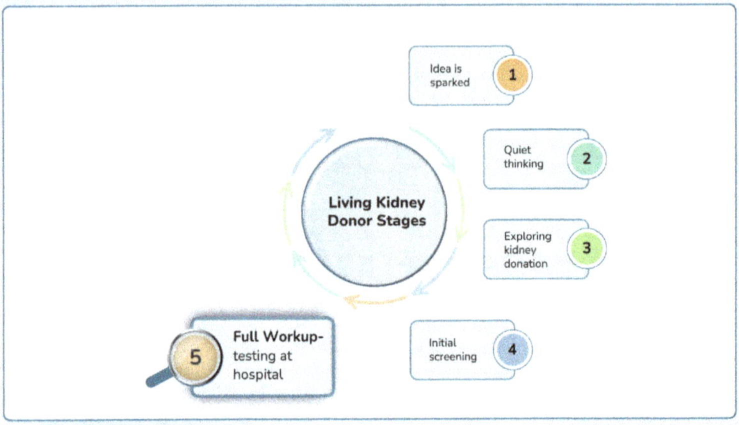

The testing for donors is paid for by the recipient's insurance. If the recipient is not known, the transplant hospital will provide the test at no cost to the donor. Later, once the recipient is identified, the recipient's insurance will cover the charges.

Some tests required for donation, like current cancer screenings (cervical, breast, prostate, colon, lung) as per the American Cancer Society or the U.S. Preventive Services Task Force guidelines, may be done outside the transplant center. If the recommended tests for the age and sex of the potential donor have already been completed, the results can be submitted. Otherwise, they can be ordered by a primary care provider, with billing typically covered by the donor's personal insurance. Once completed, the results should be submitted to the transplant center. Some donors choose to initiate this testing even before meeting with the donor coordinator, which can help expedite the workup process.

Often, bloodwork and urine tests may be done locally, if the donor does not live near the transplant center. It is important to indicate that these tests should be billed to the transplant center and not the donor's insurance. Some transplant centers send donors blood and urine containers that are to be filled locally and sent back in the prepaid mailer. Donors will be provided with a billing number to use throughout the donation process and afterward for about two years. If any billing problems occur, contact the transplant center for assistance.

When the testing is scheduled at the transplant center, the days of testing can be exhausting. Taking a friend or family member for appointments is beneficial. Some centers require a caregiver for the evaluation, pre-op, and recovery appointments. Support people can help navigate the tests, listen to the information, take notes, supply food, keep things organized, and provide general support. Some transplant centers will schedule these appointments for one to three days and others will spread them out over more time. The test results should be provided to the donor in a timely manner. The results are typically known by the transplant team within a week. The donor coordinator may need to be contacted for the results or there may be the option of viewing them in an electronic patient portal.

Sprinkled throughout the tests will be meetings with the members of the living donor team. Refer to Appendix 4 for an overview of the key roles that are essential in supporting and coordinating the donation process.

The medical evaluation requirements for living donors can be found in Appendix 5, and the psychosocial evaluation requirements for living donors can be found in Appendix 6. The medical evaluation must be performed by a physician or surgeon experienced in living donation. Note there is a general medical evaluation for all living donors (regardless of the organ) and a medical evaluation specific for living kidney donors. The psychosocial evaluation must be performed by a psychiatrist, psychologist, master's prepared social worker, or licensed clinical social worker. These requirements are based on the Organ Procurement and Transplantation Network (OPTN) policies. Additional tests may be ordered based on the results, specific health issues, or concerns. Centers must obtain living donor consent to obtain and store a blood specimen for ten years to be used only for investigating potential donor-derived diseases.

Transplant centers may intentionally delay communication with potential donors, expecting donors to initiate contact for the next step. This practice might be a way to test the donor's commitment to donating, but it is often not directly communicated to them. As a result, some donors are left wondering why they haven't received information and may mistakenly believe they have been denied the opportunity to donate, leading them to discontinue the process. A more effective approach would be for the donor team to be transparent about communication expectations.

Transplant centers may require non-directed donors to have a waiting period or "cool down" between acceptance and scheduling surgery. The period, which can be two weeks or longer depending on the center, may not always be communicated to donors. The goal is to protect the donor from making a rushed decision and to allow time to process the information from the evaluation. While this can be beneficial for some donors, it may not be necessary for everyone. Some believe that a mandatory waiting period for all non-directed donors is paternalistic and can cause unnecessary delays in providing a much-needed kidney transplant.

The multidisciplinary living donor team forms the selection committee, meeting regularly to discuss all potential donors. The goal is to ensure that a kidney is donated by someone who can live a healthy life with one kidney, although unknown risks may still exist. The frequency of these meetings varies by center, but they often occur weekly. During these meetings, workup results are reviewed to determine if:

- More testing is needed
- The donor is not a good candidate
- The donor is accepted to donate

Common additional tests might include an echocardiogram. Lifestyle changes such as lowering blood pressure or weight loss may be required. If a donor is deemed unsuitable, they may seek evaluation at another transplant center with different policies. However, sometimes it is in the donor's best interest not to donate.

The potential donor must be informed that they can decline to donate at any time.

The exact reason for canceling the donation is not shared with the recipient.

Once a donor is accepted and the recipient is ready, a surgery date can be planned. Donors are typically allowed to choose a date that suits their schedule. The donor coordinator should be informed about any blockout dates, such as work, vacation, family commitments, or any personal business, to avoid scheduling conflicts. It could be four or more weeks until surgery is scheduled. During this time, donors may feel very protective of the kidney they will be donating. They may drive under the speed limit and take extra precautions to ensure nothing happens to it before surgery. They become hyper-focused on protecting the kidney, as the worse outcome would be not being able to donate.

Sometimes the health of the recipient will delay the surgery for many months, even though the donor is ready. The chosen date must work for the donor, donor surgeon, recipient, recipient surgeon, and operating room teams.

Many tests and meetings are beyond the donor's control and can take longer than expected, causing frustration for both donors and recipients. Here are some reasons the surgery might be delayed:

- Recipient is not ready due to incomplete workup, illness, or infection.
- Recipient is not yet matched, especially for a non-directed donor or paired exchange.
- A kidney chain is being coordinated among transplant centers.
- Scheduling conflicts with the surgeon or surgery team.

- COVID-19 issues in the community.
- Weather or natural disasters.

Maintaining a healthy mind and body before surgery can aid in recovery. During the waiting time, donors can engage in supportive activities such as:

- Exercise
- Meditation/Guided imagery
- Cleaning/Organizing
- Massage
- Energy work (Reiki, Healing Touch, Reflexology, etc.)
- Yoga

If a year passes after the initial workup, some tests may have to be repeated to ensure the donor is still medically and psychologically fit to donate. The donor selection committee and the donor must both agree to proceed with the surgery. Everyone must work together to ensure a smooth process for the kidney donation.

Insights for the Chapter: Full Workup

- The living kidney donor evaluation requirements are highly regulated.
- The donor evaluation includes detailed medical and psychosocial assessments.
- Donors may decline to donate at any time.

Life is either a daring adventure or nothing.

~Helen Keller

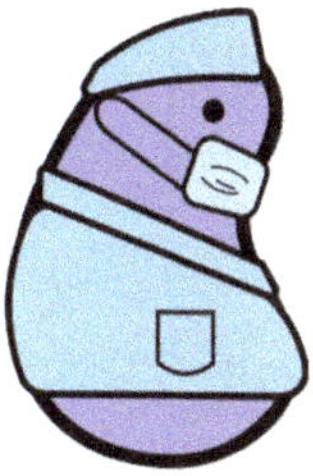

STAGE 6: SURGERY

The long-awaited day is drawing near. Preparing for surgery involves a pre-surgical visit, packing for the hospital, final preparations before the procedure, and the day of surgery itself.

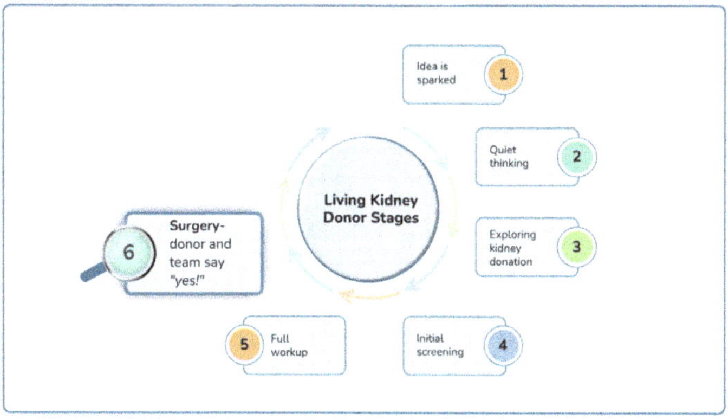

Preparation for Surgery

Once the surgery date is set, about a week before surgery, a pre-surgical visit will be scheduled. For those traveling for surgery, this visit may be the day before surgery. The primary caregiver who will be with the donor during and after surgery is required to attend.

This is a time to ask questions about the surgery, the hospital stay, and the post-op recovery plan. Final testing will be done for tissue compatibility, COVID-19, and suspected infections. There will be a review of medical information and medications.

This visit includes a meeting with the surgeon, anesthesia doctor, nephrologist, and donor coordinator to discuss final details of the surgery. The social worker and the Independent Living Donor Advocate should be available.

The surgeon will discuss the type of incision and which kidney will be removed. The left kidney is typically preferred due to the longer renal vein. There are some cases where the right kidney is removed. If both kidneys are **not** equally healthy, the better kidney is left with the donor. The type of incision can vary, depending on the surgeon, the donor's anatomy, and sometimes donor preference. A laparoscopic procedure is the most common, often including a hand-assist or robotic assist technique, and is considered minimally invasive with a quicker recovery time. This involves two small incisions (about one inch each) and one longer incision (about three to five inches) on the abdomen. Some donors require the more invasive open kidney removal with an incision up to 12 inches long on one side of the body. Prior surgeries, such as a

C-section, can affect the incision plan. If the donor would like a picture to be taken of their kidney, they should ask the surgeon. Many donors don't know this is an option and later regret not asking for a picture. (Refer to image "Living Donor Kidney.")

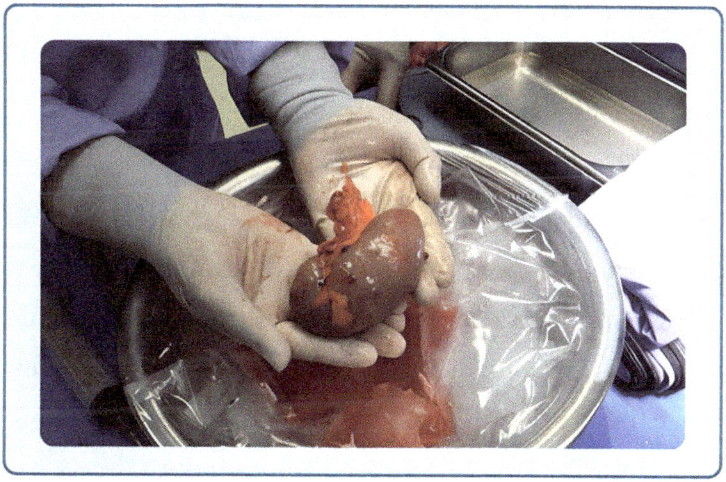

Living Donor Kidney (Zuber)

Information will be provided about when and where to come to the hospital before surgery, how the team will talk with family members, and what happens after surgery. The informed consent may also be signed at this time. The team will reinforce that the donor can back out of the surgery at any time up to the point of anesthesia; in this case, the team will disqualify them and the recipient will not be provided any details. Many donors find this reassuring. Donors should never feel pressured to follow through with donation.

The Independent Living Donor Advocate may also be present to ensure the donor's rights are protected, respected, and maintained. Questions or concerns about donating can be discussed at this time.

Information about what to eat and drink the day before surgery and when to stop eating and drinking will be provided. Placing this information in a calendar can help the donor remember these details later.

Some donors may have a bowel preparation the day before surgery, depending on the surgeon and hospital protocol. This involves taking a laxative medication and restricting the diet to help clear the colon of stool, which may lessen discomfort and ease the first bowel movement after surgery. The donor coordinator will provide the specific directions if this is ordered. Additionally, starting a stool softener before surgery might be beneficial for donors at high risk for constipation.

Donors often want to know what to pack for the hospital stay, so here is a list of items that other donors have recommended. See Table "Packing for the Hospital."

Due to COVID-19, there may be special instructions for getting a COVID test on the day of surgery. The results for the donor and recipient will be obtained before going to the operating room.

Packing for the Hospital

Clothes	Comfortable, soft loose pants, tops, socks; Clean underwear; Robe; Slippers or slide on shoes
Toiletries	Lip balm; Hand sanitizer; Lotion; Dry shampoo; Face wipes; Menstrual pads (due to stress, women may unexpectedly start their period)
Comfort	Pillow; Eye Mask; Ear plugs; Abdominal binder (request at hospital); Heating pad (request at hospital); Neck pillow; Soft blanket
Entertainment	Phone; Extra long phone charger cord; Books, magazines, eReader; Journal
Other	Insulated straw cup (request at hospital); Stool softener (request at hospital); Sense of humor; Request for a picture of the removed kidney

In the pre-operative area, there will be a final medical check and confirmation that the donor still wants to proceed, and then an IV will be started. The anesthesia doctor and the surgeon will confirm the plan for the operation. The side of the kidney to be removed will be confirmed and marked on the body. Any final questions can be asked at this time.

Remember, donors can change their mind and stop the donation up until the time of anesthesia. The living donor team will disqualify the donor, and the recipient will not be told the reason.

Surgery

Surgery often lasts around four hours, but could be longer. The donor team will update the waiting family or friends during and after surgery. The donor is taken to surgery before the recipient so the team can begin the process of removing the kidney. Later, the recipient will go into a different operating room and be prepared to receive the kidney. Often, both donor and recipient will be in the same hospital. Sometimes, the donor and the recipient will be in different hospitals and may even be in different states. In such cases, the kidney is carefully packaged for travel and taken directly to the transplant center or to an airplane to be flown to where the recipient is.

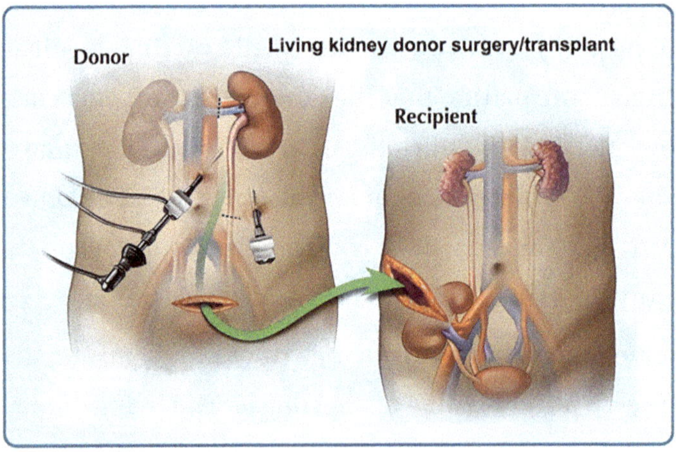

Living Kidney Donor Surgery/Transplant (Mayo)

A general anesthetic is used so nothing is felt during the surgery. Once the kidney is removed and examined, it is taken to the recipient and transplanted. Typically, the kidney from a living donor starts working right away, making urine for the recipient and immediately cleaning the blood of waste and toxins. (Refer to image "Living Kidney Donor Surgery/Transplant.")

After Surgery

Immediately after surgery, the donor is moved to the recovery room for a few hours until they begin to wake up. Typically, donors come out of surgery with:

- An oxygen tube in the nose
- IVs in the arm for fluids and pain medication
- A catheter in the bladder to collect urine
- Pressure cuffs on both legs to help prevent blood clots
- A bandage covering the new incisions where the kidney was removed; there may be one larger incision and a few smaller ones, depending on the exact surgical technique

Nurses in the recovery room will monitor blood pressure, heart rhythm, and pain level, and provide any needed medications. The surgeon will meet with the family to discuss how the surgery went, the status of the kidney, the plan for recovery, and when they can see the donor.

Insights for the Chapter: Surgery

- The type of incision will depend on the surgeon and unique aspects of the donor.
- Donors may decline to donate at any time before receiving anesthesia

Self-care means giving yourself permission to pause.

~Cecilia Tran

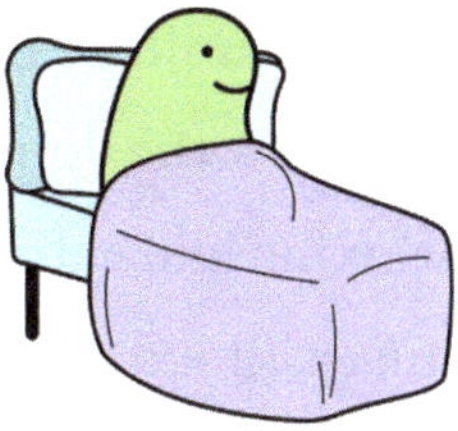

Stage 7: Recovery

The recovery stage begins in the hospital and continues at home.

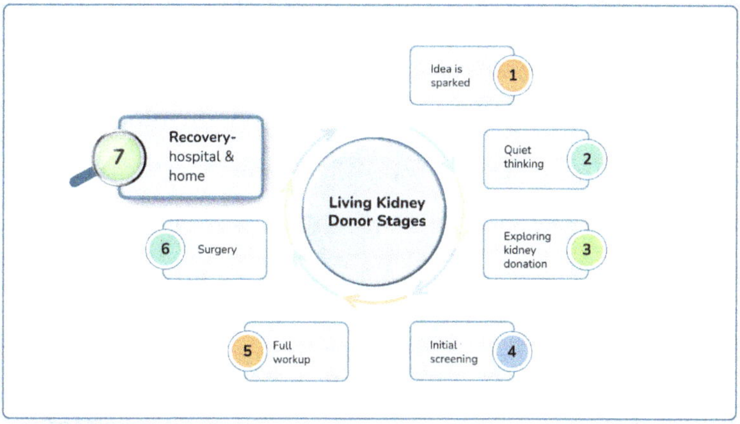

Hospital

After recovering from anesthesia, the donor is moved to a hospital room. The staff will monitor the donor for pain, any potential complications, and kidney function. It is important for the donor to resume mobility and walk to prevent possible adverse effects from the anesthesia on the body. On the first day, nurses and aides will assist the donor in getting out of bed and sitting in a chair. Drinking and eating are typically allowed if there is no nausea. Blood pressure, oxygen levels, and urine output from the remaining kidney are monitored, and comfort measures such as warm blankets, pillows for positioning, and a heating pad are provided.

Many people are concerned about pain after kidney donation surgery. The level of pain may vary depending on prior surgical experiences, the type of incision, and other factors. Generally, the pain from donating a kidney is similar to that of typical laparoscopic surgery, such as gallbladder or appendix removal. Nurses will provide pain medication to minimize discomfort. Often, a patient controlled analgesia (PCA) pump is used. An IV connected to the arm delivers pain medication rapidly through the veins, and the donor can push a button whenever more medication is needed. This eliminates the need to call and wait for the nurse to give the medication. Controlling the pain is important to encourage the donor to resume activities; otherwise, they may be reluctant to move out of bed.

It is crucial to walk several times a day to help prevent complications such as pneumonia and blood clots and to expel gas from the surgery. A small breathing device called an incentive spirometer may be used to encourage taking slow, deep breaths and to keep the lungs clear. The carbon dioxide gas used in the laparoscopic surgery can irritate the diaphragm, which may cause pain in the upper abdomen and shoulder area, especially the day after surgery.

As recovery progresses, the tubes will be removed and IV pain medications will be switched to taking pills by mouth. The catheter will be removed, and urine output will continue to be monitored. If more recovery time is needed, the hospital stay will be extended; otherwise, the donor will be discharged. Living kidney donors typically stay two to three days in the hospital. Before leaving the hospital, it is important to obtain any needed medications such as pain medication, stool softener, acetaminophen, or other prescriptions.

If the donor has traveled for the surgery, they may stay a few nights in a hotel or with family or friends before returning home. Those who have traveled by airline for the surgery may need to delay their return even longer, until they are further along in their recovery or have completed their first follow-up visit with the doctor. Some donors choose to stay with family or friends, while others may opt for a hotel or a low-cost accommodation offered by the transplant center.

Home

Proper care and management at home are crucial for a continued smooth recovery. Below is an overview of what to expect in the days and weeks following the procedure, including guidelines for pain management, mobility, and general post-operative care.

Typically, the dressing can be removed and showering is allowed after leaving the hospital. If there is drainage at the incision, a small bandage may be applied. Surgeons often use dissolvable stitches that do not need to be removed. Steri strips are often placed across the incision lines and are to be kept in place until they fall off naturally or may be removed in a couple of weeks. As the body heals, the belly may feel swollen and bloated, but this usually resolves within days or weeks. Showers may be allowed one to two days after surgery, and specific, personal instructions will be provided by the healthcare team.

It may be helpful to fill prescriptions for pain medication in advance so they are available if needed to manage pain. For many donors, only over-the-counter pain medication, such as acetaminophen, is needed by the end of the first week. It is advised that kidney donors avoid over-the-counter medications that contain nonsteroidal anti-inflammatory drugs (NSAIDs), such as aspirin and ibuprofen. This is based on the recommendation to avoid NSAIDs for people with chronic kidney disease. While there are no specific studies on NSAID use in living kidney donors, and some centers may allow NSAID use with normal kidney function as long as it is not used daily or in high doses, it is best to discuss NSAID use with healthcare providers first.

During this recovery period, feeling very tired and taking naps throughout the day is normal. Getting in and out of bed may be more difficult due to the incision, though walking up and down stairs is typically manageable. Activities will generally be at a slower pace while healing. The body takes time to clear anesthesia and for the remaining kidney to adjust to performing the functions of both kidneys. Initially, donors may have a reduced appetite, but this should return to normal with time. The body requires time to heal from the inside, even after the external incision has healed.

There will generally be a lifting limit, typically not over 10 pounds, for the first six weeks after surgery. This means there may need to be changes or accommodations made for childcare, housework, job duties, and exercise during this period. Kidney donors are advised to avoid contact sports to minimize potential harm to the remaining kidney.

Driving should be avoided for about two weeks. Most donors return to work within four to six weeks after surgery, though some may return as soon as two weeks, while others may need an additional one or two months for recovery.

It is normal to urinate more often the first few weeks after surgery. The single kidney is adjusting to performing all of the work previously done by two kidneys. Donors may find themselves getting up to urinate throughout the day and night. This pattern should normalize over time. Staying well-hydrated by drinking water throughout the day is crucial. Not enough fluid intake can place the kidney at risk for damage. Clear, pale yellow, or straw-colored urine typically indicates adequate hydration.

Body Image

Body image may be a concern for some living donors due to the changes that may occur with normal surgical trauma. During a laparoscopic procedure, CO2 gas is used to inflate the abdomen. To safely access the kidney, organs and tissues may need to be moved out of the way. This procedure creates a normal inflammatory response that requires time to heal. Abdominal bloating goes down as the gas dissipates and the inflammation decreases. Some donors' abdomens may eventually look similar to before surgery and others might experience long-lasting physical changes. Each surgeon's technique and each donor's body and lifestyle will influence recovery and appearance. The images below depict just one donor's experience.

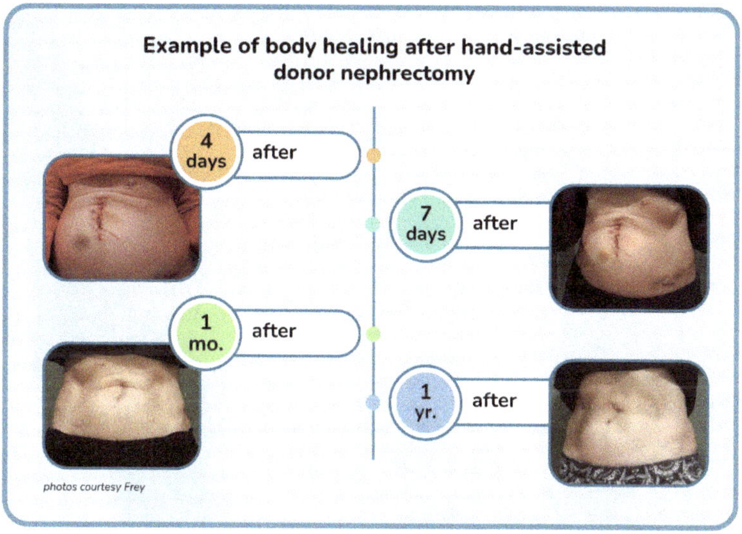

During recovery, it is important to keep the donor team informed of any problems that might arise. Contact the donor coordinator with any concerns. The goal is to eventually return to the activity level that the donor had before surgery.

Insights for the Chapter: Recovery

- Walking is important after surgery to help prevent complications.
- The typical hospital stay is two to three days.
- Frequent rest periods, modified activities, and drinking fluids is important to help the body heal at home.
- Most donors are back to work within 4-6 weeks.

Life isn't meant to be lived perfectly...
but merely to be LIVED.

Boldly, wildly, beautifully, uncertainly, imperfectly, magically LIVED.

~Mandy Hale

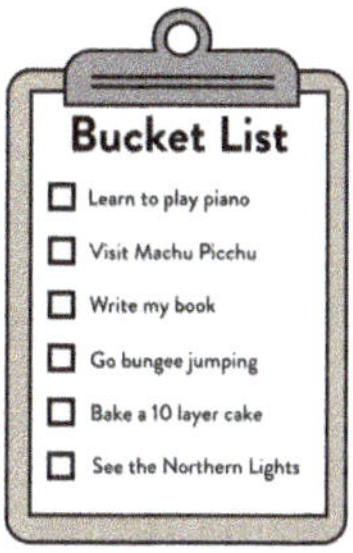

STAGE 8: FUTURE LIFE

The final stage focuses on living the rest of your life with one kidney. For most people, life after donation is not significantly different from before. Unlike recipients, donors do not need to take any new lifelong medications or follow new dietary restrictions. While excessive alcohol use is discouraged for anyone, kidney donors can consume alcohol in moderation. Donors may resume sexual activity when they feel well enough following surgery.

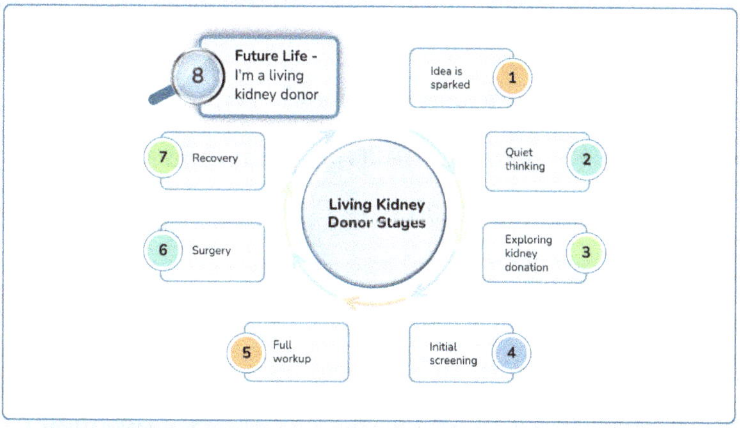

Emotional challenges can also arise. Some donors experience feelings of sadness after the surgery as they transition from the excitement of the donation process to a recovery period with physical changes. Moving from a healthy body to one that is now scarred and hurting can take an emotional toll. This shift can be emotionally challenging as they adjust to their new state of health. Additionally, stress may increase if the recipient encounters complications or if the kidney does not function as expected. In such cases, counseling can be beneficial to help cope with physical or emotional changes and the stress of daily life.

Even after recovering from the initial surgery and returning to work, the body continues to heal over the following year. Healing responses can vary widely based on factors such as prior activity level, age, the specific surgical procedure, health history, type of job, support system, and emotional well-being. It is important to keep the donor team informed of any physical or emotional symptoms.

The Organ Procurement & Transplantation Network (OPTN) policy requires follow-up reporting when the donor is discharged from the hospital and at 60 days, six months, one year, and two years post-donation. The donor team examines the surgical incision and addresses any issues within several weeks of surgery. Blood and urine are checked to evaluate kidney function and general recovery. One key indicator is the estimated glomerular filtration rate (eGFR), which measures kidney function. Normal eGFR is at least 90 ml/min per $1.73m^2$. Most donors will have a lower eGFR after donating, which is expected and may gradually return to normal over time. For some, the eGFR may remain slightly lower (less than 60 ml/min per $1.73m^2$) as a new baseline. It is important for other healthcare providers to be aware of this potential lower eGFR. The donor team should be contacted for any concerns about kidney function after donation.

Donors might notice minor physical sensations in the abdomen or upper legs from the surgery, but these typically fade over time. Major complications requiring close medical care and follow up are very rare. Some donors have reported long-term issues such as pain, nerve damage, hernia, or intestinal obstruction. Although these risks are uncommon, there are no national statistics on their frequency.

In light of the lack of data on living donors, there are some efforts to make improvements. The Chronic Disease Research Group, part of the Hennepin Healthcare Research Institute, runs the Scientific Registry of Transplant Recipients (SRTR). The SRTR created a registry to study the long-term outcomes of living organ donors called the Living Donor Collective (LDC). The mission of the LDC is to have all transplant programs across the country register all living donor candidates who come to their center for evaluation, to track the long-term outcomes of these candidates and donors. This will provide much-needed long-term data on living donors that does not currently exist.

Communicating with the Recipient

Typically, directed donors already know and talk with their recipient before and after surgery since they are often donating to family or friends. For other donors who may not have met or communicated with their recipient, there is a general process to facilitate contact.

Donors can request to reach out to their recipient through their donor coordinator before or after surgery. They may provide a card, letter, email, or other form of communication to the donor coordinator. The coordinator will then pass this information on to the recipient's transplant coordinator. It is up to the recipient to decide if they wish to respond. This process is reciprocal; if the recipient wants to contact the donor first, they follow the same procedure. Both donor and recipient must agree to communicate before any personal information (such as names, phone numbers, or email addresses) is shared.

Physical Activity

Some donors refer to donating their kidney as a "non-event." Despite the initial stress and recovery, many find that once the surgery is over and healing has occurred, the experience feels like a small incident in the context of their entire life. They often feel essentially the same as they did with two kidneys.

The goal is for donors to return to their pre-donation activity level after healing, including going back to work and resuming their favorite activities. For example, in 2022, twenty living kidney donors successfully reached the summit of Mount Kilimanjaro, the highest mountain in Africa. The organizer, Kidney Donor Athletes, has announced a three-year plan for additional One Kidney Climbs.

However, donors are advised to avoid contact sports or activities that could injure the remaining kidney. While some may experience a higher level of fatigue months or even years after surgery, most maintain an active lifestyle.

Healthy Behaviors

Regular health checkups with a primary care provider and monitoring kidney function with blood tests such as creatinine and estimated glomerular filtration rate (eGFR) are important. Many donors want to take extra precautions to stay healthy.

For some, this means being aware of drinking enough water, eating nutritious food, maintaining a healthy weight, and resuming an exercise routine. It is often advised to limit or avoid nonsteroidal anti-inflammatory drugs (NSAIDs) based on the donor team recommendations. Contrast dye that is used for imaging tests are to be used with caution, as the type and amount of dye may cause kidney damage in certain situations, especially for those with kidney disease. It is best to alert all healthcare providers about having one kidney whenever receiving medical care. Some donors have chosen to wear a medical alert bracelet indicating they have one kidney and that NSAIDs and contrast dye should be used with caution.

Women may choose to get pregnant, but should be aware of the increased risk for high blood pressure and should be monitored closely. Living kidney donors may have concerns about the risk of getting COVID-19 with one kidney. Being a kidney donor is not considered a medical condition that places one at high risk for COVID-19. The risk of getting COVID-19 is very low (around 2%) and thought to be the same for donors as for the general population.

Taking care of the body, mind, and spirit can help donors to live a long life with one kidney. Some donors like to talk about their donation story and actively promote and support living kidney donation while others only discuss donating if directly asked. Some have a strong relationship with their recipient while others don't have any or very minimal contact. Every situation is as unique as each individual donor. However, most living kidney donors have an improved quality of life and say they would donate again if they could.

Insights for the Chapter: Future Life

- Follow-up evaluations after surgery are done at 60 days, six months, one year, and two years.
- Donors do not need to take special medications or alter their diet after donating.
- Donors typically feel the same as they did with two kidneys.

Be the Change
You Wish to See
in the World

~Gandhi

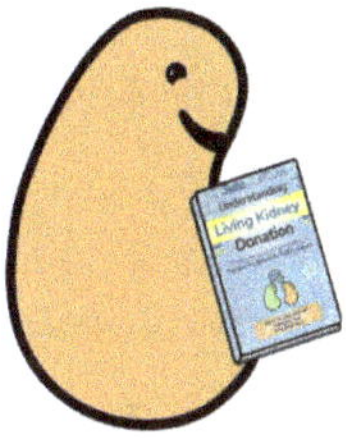

Conclusion

I began writing this book because I believed that educating more people about the benefits of living donor transplants and how to become a living kidney donor would help. I thought this could reduce the number of people on the transplant waiting list. I often say education is the answer to increasing living kidney donation because that is something I can control. However, while education is important, I no longer believe it is the sole solution.

My initial assumption was that people don't want to donate because they don't understand the process. Perhaps what I was afraid to admit is that changing society's values, laws, the medical system, and attitudes toward living donation is extremely difficult. In reality, we don't make it easy for recipients to obtain a living donor transplant or for donors to donate their kidney. Sick people (often on dialysis) are asked to go and find the best treatment: a living donor. And living donors often use their own time and money to pay for expenses related to donating.

It's time to shift legislation and prioritize living donation more than we do deceased donation because it is the best treatment for kidney failure. A national, streamlined system dedicated to living kidney donation could make it easier both for those with kidney disease and for potential donors. This would give all people on the transplant waiting list a better chance to receive a healthy living donor transplant, improve their lives, and live longer.

There Are Enough Kidneys

There are many kidneys.

Do you have two and only need one?

There are many resources.

Do you support finding living donor transplants for those with kidney disease?

Do you support those healthy enough and brave enough to donate a kidney?

There are many ways to improve efforts to discover more kidney donors.

Are you one of the millions of healthy adults who have a kidney that could be donated?

Do you support an integrated system for living donors similar to the system for deceased donors?

There are many resources and enough kidneys when we choose to break the silence and be a part of the change.

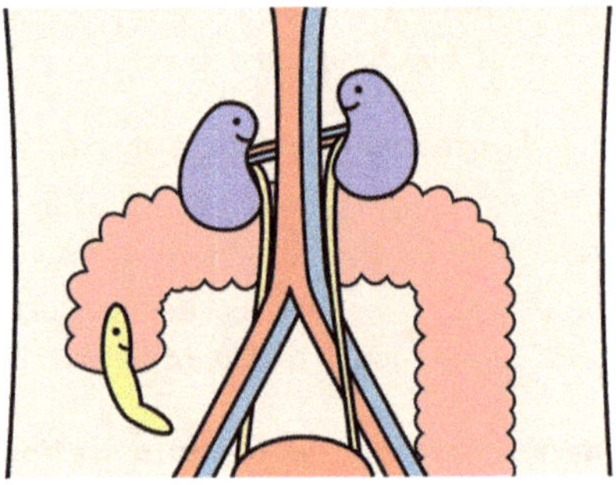

APPENDIX

APPENDIX I
CHRONIC KIDNEY DISEASE STAGES

Chronic Kidney Disease Stages

Stage	Action	Glomerular Filtration Rate (GFR)	% of Kidney Function
1	**Normal kidney function** (Healthy lifestyle)	90 or higher	90-100%
2	**Mild loss of kidney function** (Maintain normal blood pressure & blood glucose)	60-89	60-89%
3a	**Mild to moderate loss of kidney function** (See a kidney doctor)	45-59	45-59%
3b	**Moderate to severe loss of kidney function** (Begin planning for a kidney transplant & need for living kidney donor)	30-44	30-44%
4	**Severe loss of kidney function** (Initiate kidney transplant workup & have living donor start workup)	15-29	15-29%
5	**Kidney failure** (Living kidney transplant surgery)	Less than 15	Less than 15%

Appendix 2
Living Kidney Donor Risk Tools

Kidney Donor Risk Tools

Tool	Link	Estimates	Information Needed
QxMD and **ESRD Risk Tool for Kidney Donor Candidates (Chronic Kidney Disease Prognosis Consortium)**	https://qxmd.com/calculate/calculator_622/esrd-risk-tool-for-kidney-donor-candidates http://www.transplantmodels.com/esrdrisk/	• 15-year risk of end-stage kidney disease (ESKD) • Lifetime incidence of ESKD	• Age • Sex • Race • Estimated glomerular filtration rate • Systolic blood pressure • Antihypertensive medication • BMI • Diabetes history • Urine albumin to creatinine • Smoking history
Kidney Donor Risk Prediction (University of Minnesota)	https://shiny.biostat.umn.edu/Transplant/KidneyDonor/	• High blood pressure • Type 2 diabetes • Kidney function • Protein in the urine • 40-year risk of end-stage kidney disease (ESKD)	**Donor** • Age • Sex • Race • Smoking status • Estimated glomerular Filtration rate • Serum creatinine • Glucose • Body mass index • Systolic blood pressure • Diastolic blood pressure • Family history of high blood pressure • Hyperlipidemia (high blood fat levels) treated with diet/medication **Recipient** • Relationship to recipient • Recipient has type 1 diabetes • Recipient has type 2 diabetes

APPENDIX 3
LIVING KIDNEY DONATION RESOURCES

Living Kidney Donor Resources Organizations

Air Care Alliance	www.aircarealliance.org
Alliance for Paired Kidney Donation	www.paireddonation.org
American Foundation for Donation and Transplantation	www.amfdt.org
American Kidney Fund	www.kidneyfund.org
American Living Organ Donor Fund	www.helplivingdonorssavelives.org
American Society of Transplantation	www.livedonortoolkit.com
American Transplant Foundation	www.americantransplantfoundation.org
Donate Life America	www.donatelife.net
Donor Care Network	www.donorcarenet.org

Living Kidney Donor Resources Organizations

Help Hope Live	www.helphopelive.org
Health Resource and Services Administration (HRSA)	www.organdonor.gov
Kidney Donor Conversations	www.MyKDC.org
Living Donors Online	www.livingdonorsonline.org
Living Kidney Donors Network	www.lkdn.org
National Institute of Diabetes and Digestive and Kidney Diseases	www.niddk.nih.gov/health-information/kidney-disease
National Kidney Donation Organization	www.nkdo.org
National Kidney Foundation	www.kidney.org
National Kidney Registry	www.kidneyregistry.org

Living Kidney Donor Resources Organizations

National Living Donor Assistance Center	www.livingdonorassistance.org
Organ Procurement and Transplantation Network	www.optn.transplant.hrsa.gov
Scientific Registry of Transplant Recipients (SRTR)	www.srtr.org
The Transplant Journey	www.transplantjourney.org/resources
TransplantFirst Academy	www.transplantfirst.org
TransplantLyfe	www.transplantlyfe.com
United Network for Organ Sharing	www.unos.org
US Department of Health and Human Services	www.hhs.gov
WaitList Zero	www.waitlistzero.org

Living Kidney Donor Resources Community Specific

Kidney Donor Athletes	www.kidneydonorathletes.org
Kidneys for Communities	www.kidneysforcommunities.org
Living Kidney Donation for Veterans (DOVE)	www.dovetransplant.org
Modify NOTA	www.modifynota.org
Multicultural Miracle Donor Foundation	www.mmdfoundation.com
One Kidney Clubs	www.onekidneyclubs.com
Renewal	www.renewal.org

Living Donor Resources Books

- In Pursuit of a Better Life: The Ultimate Guide for Finding Living Kidney Donors by Risa Simon (2024)
- Kidney to Share by Martha Gershun & John D. Lantos (2021)
- Lost in Transplantation: Memoir of an Unconventional Organ Donor by Eldonna Edwards (2014)
- Sydney's Kidney Adventure: Her "Big Wish" for Mom Comes True! by Risa Simon (2024)
- The Fear Factor: How One Emotion Connects Altruists, Psychopaths, & Everyone In-Between by Abigail Marsh (2017)
- The Insider's Guide to Living Kidney Donation: Everything You Need to Know If You Give (or Get) the Greatest Gift by Carol Offen & Elizabeth Craig (2021)
- The Kidney Donor's Journey: 100 Questions I Asked Before Donating My Kidney by Ari Sytner (2016)
- The Organ Shortage Crisis in America: Incentives, Civic Duty, and Closing the Gap by Andrew Michael Flesher (2018)
- When Altruism Isn't Enough: The Case for Compensating Kidney Donors edited by Sally Satel (2008)

Living Kidney Donor Resources Facebook and Podcasts

Facebook	Gift of Life A Living Kidney Donor Group	facebook.com/groups/LivingKidneyDonorsRock
	Living Donor Awareness	facebook.com/groups/LivingDonorAwareness
	Living Donors with Complications	facebook.com/groups/967471196598974
	Living Kidney Donors Support Group	facebook.com/groups/2246296390
Podcasts	Donor Diaries	donordiaries.com
	The Great Social Experiment	thegreatsocialexperiment.net/podcast

Appendix 4
Living Donor Team

Living Donor Team

Office Assistant	Handles phone calls, schedules appointments, and relays information between team members.
Independent Living Donor Advocate	Required role to support donors, address concerns, and ensure the donor is not coerced. Not involved in recipient evaluation or the transplant team.
Donor Coordinator	Main nurse coordinating care for the donor, including test results, questions, and overall support throughout the process. Responsibilities fall under the broad categories of screening, assessment, education, communication, coordination and documentation.
Social Worker	Assists with psychosocial issues before, during, or after surgery including pychosocial evaluation, addressing social, personal, housing, vocational, financial, and environmental supports. May assist with advanced directives. Works with financial counselor.
Financial Counselor	Explains billing for tests, addresses insurance questions, and manages interactions with insurance companies, admissions, and billing processes.
Donor Nephrologist	Kidney specialist assessing donor kidney function, separate from the recipient's nephrologist.
Donor Surgeon	Performs kidney removal surgery, determines surgical approach, and may facilitate donor preferences during surgery (e.g., picture of kidney, music, guided imagery, etc.).
Dietician	Provides dietary guidance and support for the donor before and after surgery.
Pharmacist	Offers medication management and advice related to the donation.

Appendix 5
Medical Evaluation for All Living Donors and Living Kidney Donors

General Medical Evaluation for All Living Donors

Donor History

- Significant medical conditions
- History of infections
- Medications
- Allergies
- Coronary artery disease

Family History

- Coronary artery disease
- Cancer

Social History

- Occupation
- Employment status
- Health insurance status
- Living arrangements
- Social support
- Smoking, alcohol, and drug use and abuse
- Psychiatric illness, depression, suicide attempts
- Risk criteria for acute HIV, HBV, and HCV infection

Physical Exam

- Height, weight, body mass index (BMI)
- Vital signs
- All major organ systems

Lab and Imaging Tests

- Complete blood count (CBC) with platelet count
- Blood type and subtype
- Prothrombin Time (PT) or International Normalized Ratio (INR)
- Partial Thromboplastin Time (PTT)
- Electrolytes, blood urea nitrogen (BUN), creatinine, transaminase, albumin, calcium, phosphorus, alkaline phosphatase, bilirubin
- Pregnancy test
- Chest x-ray
- Electrocardiogram (ECG)

General Medical Evaluation for All Living Donors

Transmissible Disease Screening

- Cytomegalovirus (CMV)
- Epstein Barr Virus (EBV)
- Human Immunodeficiency Virus (HIV)
- Hepatitis B (HBV) and Hepatitis C (HCV)
- Syphilis
- Tuberculosis

Endemic Transmissible Diseases

- Hospital defines testing needed

Cancer Screening

- Cervical
- Breast
- Prostate
- Colon
- Lung

Medical Evaluation Specific to Living Kidney Donors

Kidney-Specific Donor History	• Genetic renal diseases • Kidney disease, proteinuria, hematuria • Kidney injury • Diabetes • Kidney stones • Urinary tract infections
Kidney-Specific Family History	• Kidney disease • Diabetes • Kidney cancer
Social History	• Occupation • Employment status • Health insurance status • Living arrangements • Social support • Smoking, alcohol, and drug use and abuse • Psychiatric illness, delpression, suicide attempts • Risk criteria for acute HIV, HBV, and HCV infection
Physical Exam	• Blood pressure on at least two different occasions or 24-hour or overnight blood pressure monitoring
Other Metabolic Testing	• Fasting blood glucose • Fasting lipid profile • Glucose tolerance test or glycosylated hemoglobin (HbA1c)

Medical Evaluation Specific to Living Kidney Donors

Kidney-Specific Tests

- Urinalysis
- Urine culture
- Urinary protein and albumin excretion
- Glomerular filtration rate (GFR) by isotopic method or 24-hour urine
- Hospital specific protocol for inherited kidney disease based on family history
- History of kidney stones requires a 24-hour urine stone panel

Anatomic Assessment

Determine:

- Whether the kidneys are of equal size
- If the kidneys have masses, cysts, or stones
- If the kidneys have other anatomical defects
- Which kidney is more anatomically suited for transplant

Appendix 6
Psychosocial Evaluation for Living Donors

Psychosocial Evaluation for Living Donors

Psychosocial Issues	• Mental health issues that might complicate recovery and identify risks for poor psychosocial outcome
Risk Criteria	• HIV, HBV, HCV infection
Donor History	• Smoking • Alcohol • Drug use • Substance abuse disorder
Identification of factors needed prior to the final donation decision	• Education • Therapeutic intervention
Determination of donor understanding	Short and long term medical and psychosocial risks for: • Donor • Recipient
Assessment of the decision to donate	• Free of inducement, coercion, and other undue pressure • Reasons for donating • Nature of the relationship to transplant candidate

Psychosocial Evaluation for Living Donors

Assessment of donor's ability

- Make informed decision
- Cope with major surgery and related stress
- Realistic plan for donation and recovery
- Social, emotional, financial support

Review

- Occupation
- Employment status
- Health insurance status
- Living arrangements
- Social support

Determination of understanding

- Potential financial implications of living donation

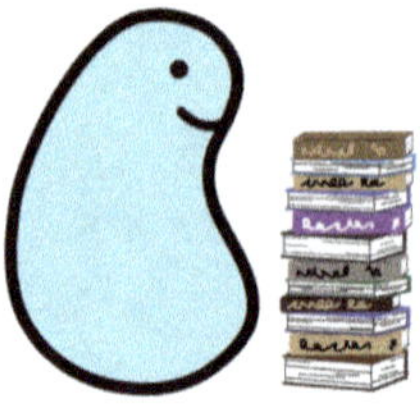

References

Introduction

American Cancer Society. "Cancer Facts & Figures 2024." Accessed December 14, 2024. https://www.cancer.org/content/dam/cancer-org/research/cancer-facts-and-statistics/annual-cancer-facts-and-figures/2024/2024-cancer-facts-and-figures-acs.pdf.

CDC: Centers for Disease Control and Prevention. "Chronic Kidney Disease in the United States, 2023." May 6, 2024. https://www.cdc.gov/kidney-disease/php/data-research/?CDC_AAref_Val=https://www.cdc.gov/kidneydisease/publications-resources/ckd-national-facts.html.

Chen, Teresa K., Daphne H. Knicely, and Morgan E. Grams. "Chronic Kidney Disease Diagnosis and Management." *JAMA* 322, no. 13 (2019): 1294–1304. https://doi.org/10.1001/jama.2019.14745.

Fishbane, Steven, and Vinay Nair. "Opportunities for Increasing the Rate of Preemptive Kidney Transplantation." *Clinical Journal of the American Society of Nephrology* 13, no. 8 (2018): 1280–82. https://doi.org/10.2215/CJN.02480218.

Lentine, Krista L., Stephen Pastan, Sumit Mohan, Peter P. Reese, Alan Leichtman, Francis L. Delmonico, Gabriel M. Danovitch, et al. "A Roadmap for Innovation to Advance Transplant Access and Outcomes: A Position Statement from the National Kidney Foundation." *American Journal of Kidney Diseases* 78, no. 3 (2021): 319–32. https://doi.org/10.1053/j.ajkd.2021.05.007.

National Kidney Foundation. "Basic Science, Clinical Research, and Kidney Disease Treatments." September 21, 2023. https://www.kidney.org/newsletter/basic-science-clinical-research-and-kidney-disease-treatments#:~:text=Learn%20more%20about%20kidney%20disease.

Naylor, Kyla L., S. Joseph Kim, Eric McArthur, Amit X. Garg, Megan K. McCallum, and Gregory A. Knoll. "Mortality in Incident Maintenance Dialysis Patients versus Incident Solid Organ Cancer Patients: A Population-Based Cohort." *American Journal of Kidney Diseases: The Official Journal of the National Kidney Foundation* 73, no. 6 (2019): 765–76. https://doi.org/10.1053/j.ajkd.2018.12.011.

NMDP. "National Marrow Donor Program." Accessed December 14, 2024. https://www.nmdp.org/.

Organ Procurement and Transplantation Network. "Educational Guidance on Patient Referral to Kidney Transplantation." Accessed December 15, 2024. https://optn.transplant.hrsa.gov/resources/guidance/educational-guidance-on-patient-referral-to-kidney-transplantation/.

Srivastava, Sudhir, Eugene J. Koay, Alexander D. Borowsky, Angelo M. De Marzo, Sharmistha Ghosh, Paul D. Wagner, and Barnett S. Kramer. "Cancer Overdiagnosis: A Biological Challenge and Clinical Dilemma." *Nature Reviews Cancer* 19, no. 6 (2019): 349–58. https://doi.org/10.1038/s41568-019-0142-8.

Stokes, John. "Consequences of Frequent Hemodialysis: Comparison to Conventional Hemodialysis and Transplantation." *Transactions of the American Clinical and Climatological Association* 122 (2011): 124–36. https://pubmed.ncbi.nlm.nih.gov/21686215/.

United States Renal Data System. "2023 Annual Data Report." Accessed July 27, 2024. https://usrds-adr.niddk.nih.gov/2023/end-stage-renal-disease.

University of California San Francisco. "The Kidney Project: Statistics." Accessed July 27, 2024. https://pharm.ucsf.edu/kidney/need/statistics#:~:text=Mortality%20rates%20vary%20depending%20on.

The Big Organ Donation Myth

Aleccia, JoNel. "How Lifesaving Organs for Transplant Go Missing in Transit." *Kaiser Health News*, February 10, 2020. khn.org/news/how-lifesaving-organs-for-transplant-go-missing-in-transit/.

Araújo, Joana, Jianwen Cai, and June Stevens. "Prevalence of Optimal Metabolic Health in American Adults: National Health and Nutrition Examination Survey 2009–2016." *Metabolic Syndrome and Related Disorders* 17, no. 1 (2019): 46–52. https://doi.org/10.1089/met.2018.0105.

Chon, W. J., M. A. Josephson, E. J. Gordon, Y. T. Becker, P. Witkowski, D. J. Arwindekar, A. Naik, J. R. Thistlethwaite, Jr., C. Liao, and L. F. Ross. "When the Living and the Deceased Cannot Agree on Organ Donation: A Survey of US Organ Procurement Organizations (OPOs)." *American Journal of Transplantation* 14, no. 1 (2013): 172–77. https://doi.org/10.1111/ajt.12519.

Cooper, Matthew, Richard Formica, John Friedewald, Ryutaro Hirose, Kevin O'Connor, Sumit Mohan, Jesse Schold, David Axelrod, and Stephen Pastan. "Report of National Kidney Foundation Consensus Conference to Decrease Kidney Discards." *Clinical Transplantation* 33, no. 1 (2018): e13419. https://doi.org/10.1111/ctr.13419.

Donate Life America. "National Donate Life Living Donor Registry." Accessed July 28, 2024. https://donatelife.net/donation/donor-registries/living-donor-registry/.

Mohan, Sumit, Mariana C. Chiles, Rachel E. Patzer, Stephen O. Pastan, S. Ali Husain, Dustin J. Carpenter, Geoffrey K. Dube, R. John Crew, Lloyd E. Ratner, and David J. Cohen. "Factors Leading to the Discard of Deceased Donor Kidneys in the United States." *Kidney International* 94, no. 1 (2018): 187–98. https://doi.org/10.1016/j.kint.2018.02.016.

Mone, Thomas, and Gabriel Danovitch. "US Organ Procurement Organization Donation Principles, Laws, and Practices." *American Journal of Kidney Diseases* 76, no. 5 (2020): 735–38. https://doi.org/10.1053/j.ajkd.2020.05.022.

National Academies of Sciences, Engineering, and Medicine. "New Report Recommends Changes to U.S. Organ Transplant System to Improve Fairness and Equity, Reduce Nonuse of Donated Organs, and Improve the System's Overall Performance." February 25, 2022. www.nationalacademies.org/news/2022/02/new-report-recommends-changes-to-u-s-organ-transplant-system-to-improve-fairness-and-equity-reduce-nonuse-of-donated-organs-and-improve-the-systems-overall-performance.

Organ Procurement and Transplantation Network. "HOPE Act." Accessed December 15, 2024. optn.transplant.hrsa.gov/professionals/by-topic/hope-act/.

Organ Procurement and Transplantation Network. "OPTN Policies Effective as of December 11, 2024." December 11, 2024. https://optn.transplant.hrsa.gov/media/eavh5bf3/optn_policies.pdf

United Network for Organ Sharing. "Frequently Asked Questions." Accessed December 15, 2024. unos.org/transplant/frequently-asked-questions/.

Verheijde, Joseph L., Mohamed Y. Rady, and Joan L. McGregor. "The United States Revised Uniform Anatomical Gift Act (2006): New Challenges to Balancing Patient Rights and Physician Responsibilities." *Philosophy, Ethics, and Humanities in Medicine* 2, no. 19 (2007). https://doi.org/10.1186/1747-5341-2-19.

Treatment for Kidney Failure

American Kidney Fund. "Deceased Donor Kidney Transplants." April 18, 2023. https://www.kidneyfund.org/kidney-donation-and-transplant/deceased-donor-kidney-transplants#:~:text=Deceased%20donor%20kidney%20transplants%20last.

Axelrod, David A., Mark A. Schnitzler, Huiling Xiao, William Irish, Elizabeth Tuttle-Newhall, Su-Hsin Chang, Bertram L. Kasiske, Tarek Alhamad, and Krista L. Lentine. "An Economic Assessment of Contemporary Kidney Transplant Practice." *American Journal of Transplantation* 18, no. 5 (2018): 1168–76. https://doi.org/10.1111/ajt.14702.

CDC: Centers for Disease Control and Prevention. "Water Use in Dialysis." March 26, 2024. https://www.cdc.gov/dialysis-safety/hcp/recommendations-resources/water-use-in-dialysis.html.

Chen, Teresa K., Daphne H. Knicely, and Morgan E. Grams. "Chronic Kidney Disease Diagnosis and Management." *JAMA* 322, no. 13 (2019): 1294–1304. https://doi.org/10.1001/jama.2019.14745.

Cheng, Xingxing S., Jialin Han, Jennifer L. Braggs-Gresham, Philip J. Held, Stephan Busque, John P. Roberts, Jane C. Tan, John D. Scandling, Glenn M. Chertow, and Avi Dor. "Trends in Cost Attributable to Kidney Transplantation Evaluation and Waiting List Management in the United States, 2012-2017." *JAMA Network Open* 5, no. 3 (2022): e221847. https://doi.org/10.1001/jamanetworkopen.2022.1847.

Doerr, Johanna Marie, Martin Juenemann, Anna Becker, Christian Nahrgang, Lucy Rainer, Juliane Liese, Andreas Hecker, Martin Wolter, Rolf Weimer, and Hristos Karakizlis. "Cognitive Profile of Kidney Transplant Patients and Impact of Deceased vs. Living Donor Transplantation." *Journal of Nephrology* 37 (2024): 1661–68. https://doi.org/10.1007/s40620-024-02004-8.

Flores, Francisco. *IMG_8963*, 2010, Flickr. Accessed December 15, 2024. https://www.flickr.com/photos/kitflores/albums/72157624671720948/.

Held, P. J., F. McCormick, A. Ojo, and J. P. Roberts. "A Cost-Benefit Analysis of Government Compensation of Kidney Donors." *American Journal of Transplantation* 16, no. 3 (2015): 877–85. https://doi.org/10.1111/ajt.13490.

Held, Philip J., Jennifer L. Bragg-Gresham, Thomas Peters, Glen M. Chertow, Frank McCormick, and John P. Roberts. "The Cost of Procuring Deceased Donor Kidneys: Evidence from OPO Cost Reports 2013-2017." *American Journal of Transplantation* 20, no. 4 (2019): 1087–94. https://doi.org/10.1111/ajt.15669.

Hoenich, Nicholas A., Robert Levin, and Catherine Pearce. "Clinical Waste Generation from Renal Units: Implications and Solutions." *Seminars in Dialysis* 18, no. 5 (2005): 396–400. https://doi.org/10.1111/j.1525-139x.2005.00078.x.

Jay, Colleen L., Patrick G. Dean, Ryan A. Helmick, and Mark D. Stegall. "Reassessing Preemptive Kidney Transplantation in the United States." *Transplantation* 100, no. 5 (2016): 1120–27. https://doi.org/10.1097/tp.0000000000000944.

Kidney Donor Conversations. "Understanding Living Kidney Donation." July 2, 2023. YouTube video. https://youtu.be/ng8n6VXya1A?si=bZ-oCx0_PnKlGpCB.

Kidney Donor Conversations. "Why a Kidney Transplant Won't Last Forever." July 4, 2024. YouTube video. https://youtu.be/EPocEXPTKQ4?si=1UrVOw1gSBgd0dS2.

Laupacis, Andreas, Paul Keown, Nancy Pus, Hans Krueger, Beryl Ferguson, Cindy Wong, and Norman Muirhead. "A Study of the Quality of Life and Cost-Utility of Renal Transplantation." *Kidney International* 50, no. 1 (1996): 235–42. https://doi.org/10.1038/ki.1996.307.

Loon, Ismay van, Marije E. Hamaker, Franciscus T.J. Boereboom, Muriel P.C. Grooteman, Peter J. Blankestijn, Rene M.A. van den Dorpel, Menso J. Nubé, Piet M. Ter Wee, Marianne C. Verhaar, and Michiel L. Bots. "A Closer Look at the Trajectory of Physical Functioning in Chronic Hemodialysis." *Age and Ageing* 46, no. 4 (2017): 594–99. https://doi.org/10.1093/ageing/afx006.

Matas, Arthur, Sally Satel, and Stephen Munn. "Incentives for Organ Donation: Proposed Standards for an Internationally Acceptable System." *American Journal of Transplantation* 12, no. 2 (2011): 306–12. https://doi.org/10.1111/j.1600-6143.2011.03881.x.

Mayo Clinic. "Living-Donor Kidney Transplant." June 28, 2024. https://www.mayoclinic.org/tests-procedures/living-donor-kidney-transplant/about/pac-20569323.

McCormick, Frank. Email to Glenna Frey. "Cost Comparison of Deceased Donor and Living Donor Transplants." June 27, 2024.

Meier-Kriesche, Herwig-Ulf, Akinlolu Ojo, Friedrich Port, Julie Arndorfer, Diane Cibrik, and Bruce Kaplan. "Survival Improvement among Patients with End-Stage Renal Disease: Trends over Time for Transplant Recipients and Wait-Listed Patients." *Journal of the American Society of Nephrology* 12, no. 6 (2001): 1293–96. https://doi.org/10.1681/asn.v1261293.

Modify NOTA. Accessed July 27, 2024. https://www.modifynota.org/.

National Institute of Diabetes and Digestive and Kidney Diseases. "Kidney Disease Statistics for the United States." May 2023. https://www.niddk.nih.gov/health-information/health-statistics/kidney-disease.

National Kidney Foundation. "Dialysis." January 2, 2023. https://www.kidney.org/atoz/content/dialysisinfo#effectiveness.

National Kidney Foundation. "Health Disparities." Accessed December 15, 2024. https://www.kidney.org/advocacy/legislative-priorities/health-disparities.

National Kidney Foundation. "Kidney Transplant." March 15, 2024. https://www.kidney.org/atoz/content/kidney-transplant.

National Kidney Foundation. "Race, Ethnicity, & Kidney Disease." Accessed December 15, 2024. https://www.kidney.org/atoz/content/minorities-KD#:~:text=Black%20or%20African%20Americans%20are.

Organ Procurement and Transplantation Network. "Frequently Asked Questions about Kidney Transplant Evaluation and Listing." Accessed July 27, 2024. https://optn.transplant.hrsa.gov/patients/by-organ/kidney/frequently-asked-questions-about-kidney-transplant-evaluation-and-listing/.

Organ Procurement and Transplantation Network. "National Data." Accessed December 15, 2024. https://optn.transplant.hrsa.gov/data/view-data-reports/national-data/#.

Raymond, Daniel. *Best Dialysis Center*, 2020, Flickr. Accessed December 15, 2024. www.flickr.com/photos/190485988@N06/.

Renewal.org. Accessed December 15, 2024. http://www.renewal.org.

Ross, Lainie Friedman, and J. Richard Thistlethwaite. "Gender and Race/Ethnicity Differences in Living Kidney Donor Demographics: Preference or Disparity?" *Transplantation Reviews* 35, no. 3 (2021): 100614. https://doi.org/10.1016/j.trre.2021.100614.

Semrau, Luke, and Arthur J. Matas. "A Regulated System of Incentives for Living Kidney Donation: Clearing the Way for an Informed Assessment." *American Journal of Transplantation* 22, no. 11 (2022): 2509–14. https://doi.org/10.1111/ajt.17129.

Siedlecki, A., W. Irish, and D. C. Brennan. "Delayed Graft Function in the Kidney Transplant." *American Journal of Transplantation* 11, no. 11 (2011): 2279–96. https://doi.org/10.1111/j.1600-6143.2011.03754.x.

Srivastava, Sudhir, Eugene J. Koay, Alexander D. Borowsky, Angelo M. De Marzo, Sharmistha Ghosh, Paul D. Wagner, and Barnett S. Kramer. "Cancer Overdiagnosis: A Biological Challenge and Clinical Dilemma." *Nature Reviews. Cancer* 19, no. 6 (2019): 349–58. https://doi.org/10.1038/s41568-019-0142-8.

Stokes, John. 2011. "Consequences of Frequent Hemodialysis: Comparison to Conventional Hemodialysis and Transplantation." *Transactions of the American Clinical and Climatological Association* 122 (2011): 124–36. https://pubmed.ncbi.nlm.nih.gov/21686215/.

Tonelli, M., N. Wiebe, G. Knoll, A. Bello, S. Browne, D. Jadhav, S. Klarenbach, and J. Gill. "Systematic Review: Kidney Transplantation Compared with Dialysis in Clinically Relevant Outcomes." *American Journal of Transplantation* 11, no. 10 (2011): 2093–2109. https://doi.org/10.1111/j.1600-6143.2011.03686.x.

United States Renal Data System. "2020 Annual Data Report: End Stage Renal Disease." Accessed December 15, 2024. https://usrds-adr.niddk.nih.gov/2020/end-stage-renal-disease.

United States Renal Data System. "2020 Annual Data Report: Incidence, Prevalence, Patient Characteristics, and Treatment Modalities." Accessed December 15, 2024. https://usrds-adr.niddk.nih.gov/2020/end-stage-renal-disease/1-incidence-prevalence-patient-characteristics-and-treatment-modalities.

United States Renal Data System. "2021 Annual Data Report:Incidence, Prevalence, Patient Characteristics, and Treatment Modalities." Accessed December 15, 2024. https://usrds-adr.niddk.nih.gov/2021/end-stage-renal-disease/1-incidence-prevalence-patient-characteristics-and-treatment-modalities.

United States Renal Data System. "2022 Annual Data Report." Accessed December 15, 2024. https://usrds-adr.niddk.nih.gov/2022.

Vadakedath, Sabitha, and Venkataramana Kandi. "Dialysis: A Review of the Mechanisms Underlying Complications in the Management of Chronic Renal Failure." *Cureus* 9, no. 8 (2017): e1603. https://doi.org/10.7759/cureus.1603.

Wang, Jeffrey H., and Allyson Hart. "Global Perspective on Kidney Transplantation: United States." *Kidney360* 2, no. 11 (2021): 1836–39. https://doi.org/10.34067/kid.0002472021.

Wesselman, Hannah, Christopher Graham Ford, Yuridia Leyva, Xingyuan Li, Chung-Chou H. Chang, Mary Amanda Dew, Kellee Kendall, et al. "Social Determinants of Health and Race Disparities in Kidney Transplant." *Clinical Journal of the American Society of Nephrology* 16, no. 2 (2021): 262–74. https://doi.org/10.2215/cjn.04860420.

Wolfe, Robert A., Valarie B. Ashby, Edgar L. Milford, Akinlolu O. Ojo, Robert E. Ettenger, Lawrence Y.C. Agodoa, Philip J. Held, and Friedrich K. Port. "Comparison of Mortality in All Patients on Dialysis, Patients on Dialysis Awaiting Transplantation, and Recipients of a First Cadaveric Transplant." *New England Journal of Medicine* 341, no. 23 (1999): 1725–30. https://doi.org/10.1056/nejm199912023412303.

Yeo, See Cheng, Xi Yan Ooi, and Tracy Suet Mun Tan. "Sustainable Kidney Care Delivery and Climate Change – A Call to Action." *Globalization and Health* 18, no. 1 (2022). https://doi.org/10.1186/s12992-022-00867-9.

Kidney Matching

Ehlayel, Abdulla, K'joy J. A. Simms, and Isa F. Ashoor. "Emerging Monitoring Technologies in Kidney Transplantation." *Pediatric Nephrology* 36 (2021): 3077–87. https://doi.org/10.1007/s00467-021-04929-9.

Kidney for Life. "Kidney for Life Initiative." Accessed July 27, 2024. https://www.kidneyforlife.org/.

Lehmann, Claudia, Sarah Pehnke, Antje Weimann, Anette Bachmann, Katalin Dittrich, Friederike Petzold, Daniel Fürst, Jonathan de Fallois, Ramona Landgraf, Reinhard Henschler, Tom H. Lindner, Jan Halbritter, Ilias Doxiadis, Bernt Popp, and Johannes Münch. "Extended Genomic HLA Typing Identifies Previously Unrecognized Mismatches in Living Kidney Transplantation." *Frontiers in Immunology* 14 (2023). https://doi.org/10.3389/fimmu.2023.1094862.

Poggio, Emilio D., Joshua J. Augustine, Susana Arrigain, Daniel C. Brennan, and Jesse D. Schold. "Long-Term Kidney Transplant Graft Survival—Making Progress When Most Needed." American Journal of Transplantation 21, no. 8 (2021): 2824–32. https://doi.org/10.1111/ajt.16463.

Ross, L. F. "Good Ethics Requires Good Science: Why Transplant Programs Should NOT Disclose Misattributed Parentage." *American Journal of Transplantation* 10, no. 4 (2010): 742–46. https://doi.org/10.1111/j.1600-6143.2009.03011.x.

Tambur, Anat R., and Rajdeep Das. "Can We Use Eplets (or Molecular) Mismatch Load Analysis to Improve Organ Allocation? The Hope and the Hype." *Transplantation* 107, no. 3 (2022): 605–15. https://doi.org/10.1097/tp.0000000000004307.

Ways to Donate a Kidney

Alliance for Paired Kidney Donation. Accessed January 14, 2025. https://paireddonation.org/.

Alliance for Paired Kidney Donation. "DonorProtect Benefits." Accessed January 14, 2025. https://paireddonation.org/donorprotect/.

Ashlagi, I., D. S. Gilchrist, A. E. Roth, and M. A. Rees. "Nonsimultaneous Chains and Dominos in Kidney- Paired Donation-Revisited." *American Journal of Transplantation* 11, no. 5 (2011): 984–94, https://doi.org/10.1111/j.1600-6143.2011.03481.x.

Cowan, N., H. A. Gritsch, N. Nassiri, J. Sinacore, and J. Veale. "Broken Chains and Reneging: A Review of 1748 Kidney Paired Donation Transplants." *American Journal of Transplantation* 17, no. 9 (2017): 2451–57. https://doi.org/10.1111/ajt.14343.

Guinness World Records. "Longest Kidney Transplant Chain." Accessed July 28, 2024. https://www.guinnessworldrecords.com/world-records/107374-longest-kidney-transplant-chain.

Kidney Donor Conversations. "Education & Support." Accessed January 14, 2025. https://mykdc.org/learn-about-kidney-donation/.

Kidney Donor Conversations. "Living Kidney Donation Voucher Programs." September 28, 2023. YouTube video. https://www.youtube.com/watch?v=KIzTRLkmrIU&feature=youtu.b.

LegiScan. "New York A02377 | 2023-2024 | General Assembly." Accessed July 27, 2024. https://legiscan.com/NY/bill/A02377/2023.

National Kidney Registry. Accessed January 14, 2025. https://www.kidneyregistry.com/.

National Living Donor Assistance Center. Accessed July 27, 2024. https://www.livingdonorassistance.org/.

Organ Procurement and Transplantation Network. "OPTN Policies Effective as of December 11, 2024." December 11, 2024. https://optn.transplant.hrsa.gov/media/eavh5bf3/optn_policies.pdf

Pope, Adam. "Nation's Longest Single-Site Kidney Chain Reaches 100." *UAB News*, July 28, 2018. https://www.uab.edu/news/health/item/9638-nation-s-longest-single-site-kidney-chain-reaches-100.

United Network for Organ Sharing. "Kidney Paired Donation – KPD." Accessed January 14, 2025. https://unos.org/transplant/kidney-paired-donation/.

Stage 3: Exploring Kidney Donation

American Society of Transplantation. "Living Donor Toolkit." Accessed December 16, 2024. https://www.livingdonortoolkit.com/.

Asmelash, Leah, and Saeed Ahmed. "He Wanted to Help a Neighbor. In the Process, He Became the Oldest Living Kidney Donor." *CNN*, June 9, 2019. https://www.cnn.com/2019/06/09/health/oldest-living-kidney-donor-trnd/index.html.

Berglund, Danielle M., Lei Zhang, Arthur J. Matas, and Hassan N. Ibrahim. 2018. "Measured Glomerular Filtration Rate after Kidney Donation: No Evidence of Accelerated Decay." *Transplantation* 102, no. 10 (2018): 1756–61. https://doi.org/10.1097/tp.0000000000002215.

Garg, Amit X., Immaculate F. Nevis, Eric McArthur, Jessica M. Sontrop, John J. Koval, Ngan N. Lam, Ainslie M. Hildebrand, et al. "Gestational Hypertension and Preeclampsia in Living Kidney Donors." *New England Journal of Medicine* 372, no. 2 (2015): 124–33. https://doi.org/10.1056/nejmoa1408932.

Hoyert, Donna L. "Maternal Mortality Rates in the United States, 2021." *Centers for Disease Control and Prevention*, March 16, 2023. https://stacks.cdc.gov/view/cdc/124678.

Ibrahim, Hassan N., Robert Foley, LiPing Tan, Tyson Rogers, Robert F. Bailey, Hongfei Guo, Cynthia R. Gross, and Arthur J. Matas. "Long-Term Consequences of Kidney Donation." *New England Journal of Medicine* 360, no. 5 (2009): 459–69. https://doi.org/10.1056/nejmoa0804883.

Lentine, Krista L., Ngan N. Lam, and Dorry L. Segev. "Risks of Living Kidney Donation: Current State of Knowledge on Outcomes Important to Donors." *Clinical Journal of the American Society of Nephrology* 14, no. 4 (2019): 597–608. https://doi.org/10.2215/CJN.11220918.

Lentine, Krista L., and Anita Patel. "Risks and Outcomes of Living Donation." *Advances in Chronic Kidney Disease* 19, no. 4 (2012): 220–28. https://doi.org/10.1053/j.ackd.2011.09.005.

Marsh, Abigail. *The Fear Factor: How One Emotion Connects Altruists, Psychopaths, and Everyone In-Between.* Basic Books, 2017.

Massey, Emma K., Mathilde C. Pronk, Willij C. Zuidema, Willem Weimar, Jacqueline Wetering, and Sohal Y. Ismail. "Positive and Negative Aspects of Mental Health after Unspecified Living Kidney Donation: A Cohort Study." *British Journal of Health Psychology* 27, no. 2 (2021): 374–89. https://doi.org/10.1111/bjhp.12549.

Massie, Allan B., Jennifer D. Motter, Jon J. Snyder, Macey L. Levan, and Dorry L. Segev. 2024. "Thirty-Year Trends in Perioperative Mortality Risk for Living Kidney Donors." *JAMA* 332, no. 12 (2024): 1015–17. https://doi.org/10.1001/jama.2024.14527.

McCormick, Frank, Philip J. Held, and Glenn M. Chertow. "The Terrible Toll of the Kidney Shortage." *Journal of the American Society of Nephrology* 29, no. 12 (2018): 2775–76. https://doi.org/10.1681/asn.2018101030.

Mena-Gutierrez, Alejandra M., Amber M. Reeves-Daniel, Colleen L. Jay, and Barry I. Freedman. "Practical Considerations for APOL1 Genotyping in the Living Kidney Donor Evaluation." *Transplantation* 104, no. 1 (2020): 27–32. https://doi.org/10.1097/tp.0000000000002933.

National Living Donor Assistance Center. Accessed July 27, 2024. https://www.livingdonorassistance.org/.

National Safety Council. "Odds of Dying." Accessed December 16, 2024. https://injuryfacts.nsc.org/all-injuries/preventable-death-overview/odds-of-dying/.

Organ Procurement and Transplantation Network. "OPTN Policies Effective as of December 11, 2024." December 11, 2024. https://optn.transplant.hrsa.gov/media/eavh5bf3/optn_policies.pdf
.

Przech, Sebastian, Amit X. Garg, Jennifer B. Arnold, Lianne Barnieh, Meaghan S. Cuerden, Christine Dipchand, Liane Feldman, et al. "Financial Costs Incurred by Living Kidney Donors: A Prospective Cohort Study." *Journal of the American Society of Nephrology* 29, no. 12 (2018): 2847–57. https://doi.org/10.1681/ASN.2018040398.

Renewal.org. Accessed December 15, 2024. http://www.renewal.org.

Sachdeva, Mala, Lisa M. Rosen, Jeny Varghese, Steven Fishbane, and Ernesto P. Molmenti. "Weight Trends in United States Living Kidney Donors: Analysis of the UNOS Database." *World Journal of Transplantation* 5, no. 3 (2015): 137–44. https://doi.org/10.5500/wjt.v5.i3.137.

Serur, David, Todd Pesavento, Emilio Poglio, Rebecca Hays, and Didier Mandelbrot. "Life with One Kidney: Primary Care and the Living Kidney Donor." *The American Journal of Medicine* 130, no. 7 (2017): 763–65. https://doi.org/10.1016/j.amjmed.2017.02.017.

Unalp-Arida, Aynur, and Constance E. Ruhl. "The Burden of Gallstone Disease in the United States Population." January 26, 2024. https://doi.org/10.1101/2022.07.08.22277386.

United Network for Organ Sharing. "Living Donation." Accessed December 16, 2024. https://unos.org/transplant/living-donation/.

United Network for Organ Sharing. "Theological Perspective on Organ and Tissue Donation." Accessed December 16, 2024. https://unos.org/transplant/facts/theological-perspective-on-organ-and-tissue-donation/.

University of Michigan Health. "Living Kidney Donation." Accessed July 28, 2024. https://www.uofmhealth.org/conditions-treatments/transplant/living-and-paired-kidney-donation.

Van Pilsum Rasmussen, Sarah E., Miriam Robin, Amrita Saha, Anne Eno, Romi Lifshitz, Madeleine M. Waldram, Samantha N. Getsin, et al. "The Tangible Benefits of Living Donation: Results of a Qualitative Study of Living Kidney Donors." *Transplantation Direct* 6, no. 12 (2020): e626. https://doi.org/10.1097/TXD.0000000000001068.

Wirken, L., H. van Middendorp, C. W. Hooghof, M. M. Rovers, A. J. Hoitsma, L. B. Hilbrands, and A. W. M. Evers. "The Course and Predictors of Health-Related Quality of Life in Living Kidney Donors: A Systematic Review and Meta-Analysis." *American Journal of Transplantation* 15, no. 12 (2015): 3041–54. https://doi.org/10.1111/ajt.13453.

Stage 4: Initial Screening

CMS: Centers for Medicare and Medicaid Services. "State Operations Manual: Appendix X – Guidance to Surveyors: Organ Transplant Programs." February 21, 2020, https://www.cms.gov/Regulations-and-Guidance/Guidance/Manuals/downloads/som107ap_x_otp.pdf.

DOVE Transplant. "Become a DOVE Donor." Accessed December 16, 2024. https://www.dovetransplant.org/new-donor.

Kidney Donor Conversations. Accessed December 16, 2024. https://mykdc.org/.

Kidney Transplant Centers. "Best Kidney Transplant Centers in the U.S." Accessed December 16, 2024. https://www.kidneytransplantcenters.org/.

National Kidney Donation Organization. "Considering Kidney Donation." Accessed December 16, 2024. https://www.nkdo.org/considering-kidney-donation/.

National Kidney Registry. Accessed December 16, 2024. https://www.kidneyregistry.com/.

Renewal.org. Accessed December 15, 2024. https://www.renewal.org/.

U.S. Department of Veterans Affairs. "VA National Transplant Program." April 17, 2024. https://www.va.gov/health/services/transplant/.

U.S. News & World Report. "Best Hospitals for Kidney Failure." Accessed December 16, 2024. https://health.usnews.com/best-hospitals/hospital-ratings/kidney-failure.

Stage 5: Full Workup

American Cancer Society. "American Cancer Society Prevention and Early Detection Guidelines." Accessed December 16, 2024. www.cancer.org/health-care-professionals/american-cancer-society-prevention-early-detection-guidelines.html.

Bernabe, Angeline Jane. "Kidney Donors Climb Mt. Kilimanjaro to Raise Awareness about Living Organ Donation." *Good Morning America*, March 10, 2022. https://www.goodmorningamerica.com/wellness/story/kidney donors-climb-mt-kilimanjaro-raise-awareness-living-83358786.

CDC: Centers for Disease Control and Prevention. "COVID Data Tracker." Accessed December 16, 2024. https://covid.cdc.gov/covid-data-tracker/#datatracker-home.

CMS: Centers for Medicare and Medicaid Services. "Medicare Program; Hospital Conditions of Participation: Requirements for Approval and Re-Approval of Transplant Centers to Perform Organ Transplants." *Federal Register* 72, no. 61 (2007). www.cms.gov/regulations-and-guidance/legislation/cfcsandcops/downloads/trancenterreg2007.pdf

CMS: Centers for Medicare and Medicaid Services. "State Operations Manual: Appendix X – Guidance to Surveyors: Organ Transplant Programs." February 21, 2020, https://www.cms.gov/Regulations-and-Guidance/Guidance/Manuals/downloads/som107ap_x_otp.pdf.

Doshi, Mona D., Demetra Tsapepas, Rohini Prashar, Sumit Mohan, Emmanuel Edusei, Meredith J. Aull, Eric Sherman, and Darshana M. Dadhania. "COVID-19 Infection in Former Living Kidney Donors." *Clinical Transplantation* 35, no. 4 (2021): e14230. https://doi.org/10.1111/ctr.14230.

Garg, Amit X., Immaculate F. Nevis, Eric McArthur, Jessica M. Sontrop, John J. Koval, Ngan N. Lam, Ainslie M. Hildebrand, et al. "Gestational Hypertension and Preeclampsia in Living Kidney Donors." *New England Journal of Medicine* 372, no. 2 (2015): 124–133. https://doi.org/10.1056/nejmoa1408932.

Kidney Donor Athletes. Accessed December 16, 2024. https://kidneydonorathlete.org/.

Living Donor Collective. "Who We Are." Accessed July 28, 2024. https://livingdonorcollective.org/about-ldc/who-we-are/.

Matas, Arthur J., and Hassan N. Ibrahim. "The Unjustified Classification of Kidney Donors as Patients with CKD: Critique and Recommendations." *Clinical Journal of the American Society of Nephrology* 8, no. 8 (2013): 1406–1413. https://doi.org/10.2215/cjn.02110213.

National Kidney Foundation. "Long-Term Risks of Living Donation." August 27, 2024. www.kidney.org/transplantation/livingdonors/long-term-risks.

Organ Procurement and Transplantation Network. "OPTN Policies Effective as of December 11, 2024." December 11, 2024. https://optn.transplant.hrsa.gov/media/eavh5bf3/optn_policies.pdf

Vandenberghe, Wim, and Eric Hoste. "Contrast-Associated Acute Kidney Injury: Does It Really Exist, and If So, What to Do about It?" *F1000Research* 8 (2019): 753. https://doi.org/10.12688/f1000research.16347.1.

Stage 6: Surgery

Khalil, Ali, Muhammad A. Mujtaba, Tim E. Taber, Muhammad S. Yaqub, William Goggins, John Powelson, Chandru Sundaram, and Asif A. Sharfuddin. "Trends and Outcomes in Right vs. Left Living Donor Nephrectomy: An Analysis of the OPTN/UNOS Database of Donor and Recipient Outcomes—Should We Be Doing More Right-Sided Nephrectomies?" *Clinical Transplantation* 30, no. 2 (2015): 145–53, https://doi.org/10.1111/ctr.12668.

Mayo Clinic. "Living-Donor Kidney Transplant." June 28, 2024. https://www.mayoclinic.org/tests-procedures/living-donor-kidney-transplant/about/pac-20569323.

Living Kidney Donors Support Group. "What to Bring to the Hospital." *Facebook*, July 3, 2018. https://www.facebook.com/groups/2246296390/files/files.

Zuber, Ben. *Living Donor Kidney*, June 20, 2019. Photo sent to author on June 11, 2020.

Stage 7: Recovery

Armstrong, Lawrence E., Carl M. Maresh, John W. Castellani, Michael F. Bergeron, Robert W. Kenefick, Kent E. LaGasse, and Deborah Riebe. "Urinary Indices of Hydration Status." *International Journal of Sport Nutrition and Exercise Metabolism* 4, no. 3 (1994): 265–79. https://doi.org/10.1123/ijsn.4.3.265.

Baker, Megan, and Mark A. Perazella. "NSAIDs in CKD: Are They Safe?" *American Journal of Kidney Diseases* 76, no. 4 (2020): 546–57. https://doi.org/10.1053/j.ajkd.2020.03.023.

Frey, Glenna. *1 Month after Hand Assisted Donor Nephrectomy*, May 24, 2017. Photo by author.

---. *1 Year after Hand Assisted Donor Nephrectomy*, April 24, 2018. Photo by author.

---. *4 Days after Hand Assisted Donor Nephrectomy*, April 28, 2017. Photo by author.

---. *7 Days after Hand Assisted Donor Nephrectomy*, May 1, 2017. Photo by author.

Health Resources and Services Administration. "Living Organ Donation." March 2023. https://www.organdonor.gov/learn/process/living-donation.

Li, Xinyou, and Kezhong Li. "Time Characteristics of Shoulder Pain after Laparoscopic Surgery." *Journal of the Society of Laparoscopic & Robotic Surgeons* 25, no. 2 (2021): e2021.00027. https://doi.org/10.4293/JSLS.2021.00027.

Perrier, E. T., J. H. Bottin, M. Vecchio, and G. Lemetais. "Criterion Values for Urine-Specific Gravity and Urine Color Representing Adequate Water Intake in Healthy Adults." *European Journal of Clinical Nutrition* 71, no. 4 (2017): 561–63. https://doi.org/10.1038/ejcn.2016.269.

United Network for Organ Sharing. "Living Donation." Accessed December 16, 2024. https://unos.org/transplant/living-donation/.

Stage 8: Future Life

Organ Procurement and Transplantation Network. "OPTN Policies Effective as of December 11, 2024." December 11, 2024. https://optn.transplant.hrsa.gov/media/eavh5bf3/optn_policies.pdf .

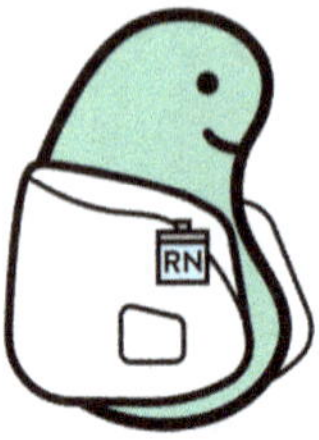

Author's Note

In the 1980s, I was a young nurse working with kidney transplant patients. Sometimes family members would donate their kidney and that seemed like a loving, logical thing to do. In later years, I was working in a dialysis unit and was told about a nurse who donated their kidney to a patient on dialysis. The idea that someone would put themselves at potential risk to help a non-relative get off dialysis was nothing short of amazing. It opened my mind and touched my heart and soul. This was the spark that would eventually lead me to donate my kidney to a complete stranger.

While I was growing up, my mother always talked about wanting to be a nurse. Finally, in her late forties, she entered school to become a licensed practical nurse. I was in high school at the time and would help her study. I remember loving anatomy and learning how complex body systems worked together. Later, I began working as an aide in a local community hospital and discovered that I loved the environment and helping the sick feel better. I graduated from Bowling Green State University with a bachelor's degree in nursing in 1981. In 1991, I returned to school and earned a master's degree in nursing as a clinical nurse specialist from the Medical College of Ohio.

What I enjoy the most about nursing is found in the first three provisions of the American Nurses Association Code of Ethics for Nurses:

- The nurse practices with compassion and respect for the inherent dignity, worth, and unique attributes of every person.
- The nurse's primary commitment is to the patient, whether an individual, family, group, community, or population.
- The nurse promotes, advocates for, and protects the rights, health, and safety of the patient.

As a nurse, my job is to prioritize the best interests of the patient, considering their unique values, preferences, and goals. This sometimes involves challenging physician orders or hospital policies. My passion is to be a strong advocate that empowers individuals, families, communities, and those with kidney disease. I want to help them make informed decisions, and support and honor them through both living and the end of life.

I was hooked on nephrology nursing even before I was a nurse. While in nursing school, I worked as a nursing assistant at the Medical College of Ohio and loved my time on the kidney transplant unit. I provided one-to-one nursing care to patients after surgery, including hourly monitoring of vital signs, kidney function, and IV fluids, all while in total isolation with gown, mask, and gloves. It was incredibly rewarding to witness patients who had been very sick recover with a functioning kidney and leave the hospital free from dialysis. After becoming a nurse, I continued working in the transplant unit and later learned to perform peritoneal dialysis and hemodialysis.

I first met my husband's family while working in that same kidney transplant unit, where his father was a patient. Several months later, I met my husband on a blind date. By then, I was aware that he and his family had polycystic kidney disease (PKD). We got married a year later, in 1985. After many discussions about the genetic implications of PKD, we eventually had two children. We knew that each child would have a 50-50 chance of receiving an autosomal dominant PKD (ADPKD) gene from him.

My husband was 43 when he received his first kidney transplant from my niece in 2002. I was blood type A and he was blood type O, so I could not donate my kidney to him. It wasn't until later that I learned about the paired kidney exchange as an option for incompatible donors and recipients. Because he was only in his forties and living donor transplants last around 20 years, that meant he would eventually need another kidney. My plan was to donate my kidney to him through a paired exchange when he needed a second transplant.

I have since discovered that very few people are planning for another transplant soon after they receive one that is working. Kidney transplants don't last forever. However, recipients and their families rarely discuss in advance how they plan to obtain another kidney and prevent dialysis.

In 2015, my husband's transplanted kidney was doing very well with no signs of rejection. On a crisp, sunny fall day in October, he had a conversation with me that would alter my kidney donation plan. I would soon be 57, and he said, "You are getting older." I was six months older than he was, so I thanked him for this observation and replied, "You are too. What's your point?" He continued, "I know you've been saving your kidney for me, but I don't need it now and you are getting older. If you want to give it away, maybe you should do it sooner rather than later and give it to someone else."

I had not even considered the fact that while I had been waiting for him to need my kidney, I was aging! Even though there is no upper age limit for donating, I knew that kidney function diminishes with age, so what he said made a lot of sense. I immediately decided to donate my kidney as soon as possible. The worst thing I could imagine was being unable to donate due to a future medical issue.

During my donor workup, I was told about a new option called the voucher program. I could donate to a stranger now and family members could receive a voucher (like a coupon) for a kidney later. If one of them develops kidney failure, they can turn in the voucher and be matched for a kidney transplant. This sounded like a great option since both my husband and daughter have PKD. My donor information was placed into the National Kidney Registry and I was matched with a stranger. In return, both my husband and daughter received vouchers. Only one of them will be able to turn theirs in for a kidney transplant. I was the first voucher donor at Cleveland Clinic, Ohio; my recipient has a working kidney and got off dialysis. And the voucher program allows me to help someone I love in the future.

Although I was a nephrology nurse, I gained even more knowledge about living kidney donation through my own experience with the process. The following year, my daughter, Amanda, and I discussed the lack of public information on living donation. While there was a movement to get people registered to be deceased donors, there was little focus on living donor transplants, which can be obtained faster and last longer. No one seemed to be discussing this and there was no support for living donors. So, in 2018, we started the nonprofit Kidney Donor Conversations. The mission of Kidney Donor Conversations is to provide education and support for living kidney donation. We offer one-on-one support, presentations, community events, videos, and written materials. Additional resources are available on our website at www.MyKDC.org and on our YouTube channel: https://www.youtube.com/@kidneydonorconversations.

My most challenging labor of love has been writing this book *Understanding Living Kidney Donation: The Best Treatment for Kidney Disease*. Donating my kidney to a stranger was easy compared to the task of helping people understand the process, options, and benefits of living kidney donation.

I discuss the voucher programs whenever I interact with potential donors or recipients. Vouchers are an excellent way to plan for anyone who may need a second or third kidney transplant in the future. Anyone healthy enough to donate can make a non-directed donation (to a stranger) and receive vouchers for loved ones. The individuals named on the voucher do not need to have kidney disease or be related to the donor. The National Kidney Registry and the Alliance for Paired Kidney Donation both offer voucher-type programs.

My husband did eventually need a second kidney transplant in 2020. Someone stepped forward to donate a kidney to him again and he did not need to use his voucher. My daughter has normal kidney function and still has her voucher. I am leading a healthy life with one kidney after donating over seven years ago. I have not met my recipient, and although I have reached out many times, they have not responded. My only regret as a living kidney donor is that I don't have more kidneys to give away so that I could save more lives.

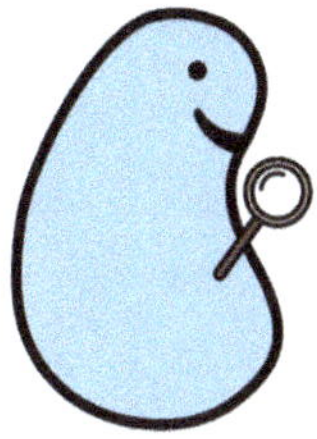

Index

E

F

G

H

K

L

M

N

O

P

S

T

Y

Z

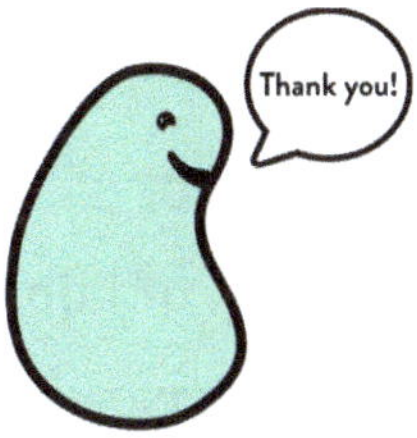

ACKNOWLEDGMENTS

All the Living Kidney Donors

Many thanks to the past and future living kidney donors. You illuminate the path for those with kidney disease and save lives through your gift of love and the best treatment—a living donor transplant.

My Volunteer Editors

I deeply appreciate all the time and effort you invested in providing me with much-needed feedback during the early stages of this book.

- Glory I. Chukwusom, MSN, APRN
- Pam Cochran
  https://www.linkedin.com/me?trk=p_mwlite_feed-secondary_nav
- Cheryl Gomez, MSN, RN, EBP(CH)
- Deb Guzman, MSN, RN

- Karen Guerra, MSW
  https://www.instagram.com/kshady8/
    - In loving memory of Jaime Guerra. My dad was on dialysis for 16 years and a transplant recipient in 2007 and 2019. This is my way of giving back to who has been in his shoes, in his donor's shoes, and mine.
- Martha Gershun www.marthagershun.com
- Jill A. Green, PhD @JillAGreen1
- Robin Glaza, DNP, MSN, RN, NPD-BC
  linkedin.com/in/drrobinglaza
- Judy Sparks Grifhorst
  https://www.facebook.com/groups/2283606491667131
- Melinda Martin Lester, RN,BA CNNe
  http://www.facebook.com/mmartinlester
- Samhita (Diya) Sengupta
- Heidi M. Shank, RN, MSN, DNP
  www.linkedin.com/in/heidi-shank-b9808238
- Rebekah Thomas
- Lara Tushla, LCSW, NSW-C
- Two additional anonymous editors

Kidney Donor Conversations, Inc.

Thank you for the nonprofit's sponsorship. I extend my gratitude to the Board of Directors for their unwavering support and patience throughout this lengthy process. A very special thanks to Dave Switzer and Tara O'Brien, PhD, RN, CNE for believing in me and helping me see this book through to the end.

Cleveland Clinic Transplant Team

Thank you for the exceptional care and support during my kidney donation journey in 2017. Your expertise and compassion made a remarkable difference. A special thanks goes to Karen Wallenfelsz, RN, my donor coordinator, and Dr. Stuart Flechner, MD, my surgeon, for their dedication and never giving up on me. I am eternally grateful to Dr. Susan B. LeGrand, MD, whose actions literally shifted my fate and made all of this possible.

My Expert Designers, Editors, and Mentor

Thank you for your guidance. Your expertise has transformed this into something uniquely polished that exceeded my expectations: Becky Meyer, Madeleine Swart, Naya Lizardo, Iqra Rafiq, and Risa Simon for your ongoing wisdom, support, and encouragement.

Videographer

Thanks to Molly Mickley, who has literally made Amanda's kidneys come to life. We love working with you, brainstorming, and watching you transform our ideas into fun images.

https://www.mollymickley.com/

ChatGPT

Thank you for being the collaborative partner that helped organize, edit, and clarify all the ideas in my head.

Canva

Thank you for being the creative designer that helped make this book more interesting and fun.

My Friends

Ann Ellis, Julie DiBacco, Robin Glaza, Cheryl Gomez, Deb Guzman, Caroline Mak, and Judy Szor. Thank you for supporting me through the ups and downs of living in a family affected by kidney disease and navigating the challenging world of healthcare as a nurse. Your love and support mean the world to me.

My Parents

Eunice Mae Lee and Glenn Howard Baumbarger. Thank you for being my role models and my legacy. Your love and desire to help others molded me into a nurse, a living kidney donor, and an author. It has been an honor to be your daughter.

My Siblings

Carol Meyer and Gary Baumbarger. Thank you for your guidance, strength, support, and loving family bond over the years. As your little sister, I have always looked up to both of you!

My Husband

Dr. Robert D. Frey. Thank you for tolerating my obsession with kidneys over all these years. What a journey this has been since our first blind date in 1984.

My Children

Sawyer Frey and Elle George Frey. Thank you for returning to Ohio with Zora! My life has blossomed and my heart is overjoyed with you close.

Chirag Thaker. Thank you for hosting my many weekend visits, tolerating our kidney discussions, and for bringing me food and coffee.

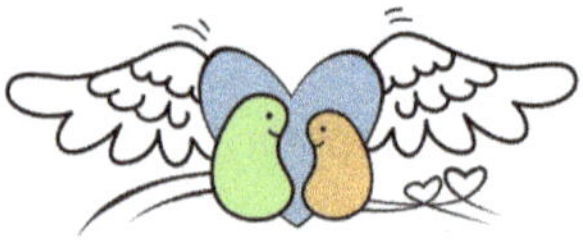

Amanda Frey. Kidney Donor Conversations wouldn't exist, and this book wouldn't have been written, without you by my side for all these years. Thank you for the adorable kidneys that help make all that we do more fun! You are the wind beneath my wings.

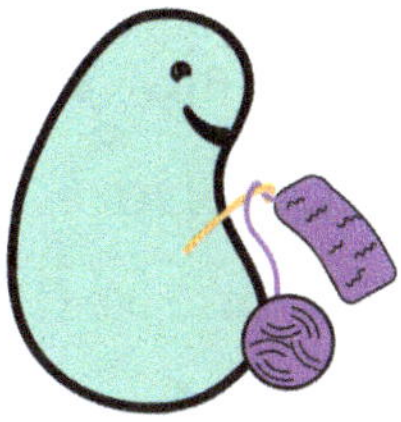

About the Author

Glenna (Baumbarger) Frey, MSN, APRN-CNS, has dedicated over 40 years to nephrology nursing, specializing in hemodialysis, peritoneal dialysis, and kidney transplantation. In 2017, she donated a kidney to a stranger at the Cleveland Clinic. The following year, she co-founded Kidney Donor Conversations (KDC), a nonprofit providing education and support for living kidney donation with her daughter, Amanda. Glenna serves as executive director of KDC and frequently presents programs on living kidney donation. She is a member of the American Nephrology Nurses Association and the National Kidney Donation Organization. She volunteers with the National Kidney Foundation and other kidney-focused groups.

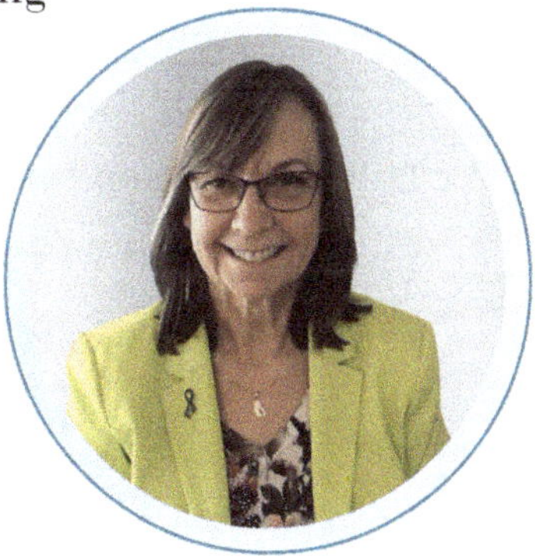

Her connection to kidney disease and transplantation is deeply personal. Many of her relatives, including her husband Bob, have Polycystic Kidney Disease (PKD). Bob has undergone dialysis and is now living with his second kidney transplant from a living donor. Her children, Amanda and Sawyer, also have PKD but currently maintain normal kidney function.

Glenna is a published author and contributor to several works on kidney donation and nephrology nursing, including *In Pursuit of a Better Life: The Ultimate Guide for Finding Living Kidney Donors, Thriving Post Kidney Transplant,* and the *Nephrology Nursing Journal.* Additionally, she served as a reviewer for the 4th edition of *Contemporary Nephrology Nursing.*

Glenna also specializes in holistic therapies, holds a Black Belt in Tae Kwon Do, and is a Hula Hoop instructor. She resides in Northwest Ohio with her husband and enjoys time with her cat, chocolate lab, as well as crocheting, and native plant gardening. Glenna's pride and joy are her children, Amanda and Sawyer, and her granddaughter, Zora.

For inquiries, contact:

https://sites.google.com/view/glennafreyauthor/home

or visit

https://www.facebook.com/LivingKidneyDonationBook

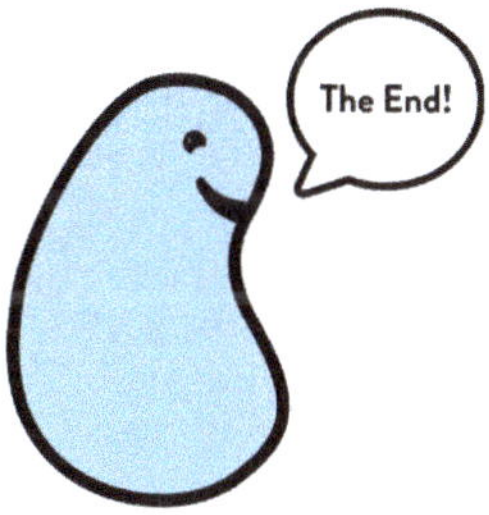
The End!

www.ingramcontent.com/pod-product-compliance
Lightning Source LLC
LaVergne TN
LVHW050812061126
851857LV00012B/771